MW01235427

"This book is a delightful read."

"I think the book is of great value"

Ranga Krishnan, M.D., Professor and Chair of Psychiatry
Duke University Medical Center

"I can't recall ever seeing a book which applied this approach to the challenge of opening the field of psychiatry to the general public."

Robert N. Golden, M.D., Professor and Chair of Psychiatry
University of North Carolina

"This book fills a void that has existed too long for both professionals and the rest of us who want to help ourselves"

Rev. Sidney L. Freeman, Ph.D.

"A magical book."

"A book of amazing stories indeed."

John M. Oldham, M.D., Professor and Chair, Department of Psychiatry
Medical University of South Carolina

"I would strongly recommend this outstanding book to people suffering from a mental illness, their caregivers, as well as care providers (physicians, psychologists, social workers) and students."

Dilip V. Jeste, M.D., Professor and Director of Ageing
VA Hospital, San Diego, California

SOLVING PSYCHIATRIC PUZZLES

by

V. SAGAR SETHI, M.D., Ph.D.
with
George W. Jacobs

1663 Liberty Drive, Suite 200
Bloomington, Indiana 47403
(800) 839-8640
www.authorhouse.com

First published by AuthorHouse 09/08/04

ISBN: 1-4184-6696-4 (sc)
ISBN: 1-4184-6695-6 (dj)

Library of Congress Control Number: 2004095214

Printed in the United States of America
Bloomington, Indiana

This book is printed on acid-free paper.

The names of all patients who are referred by first name only in this book have been disguised in name and physical description to protect their privacy.

Sethi, Vidya Sagar, 1937-
Solving Psychiatric Puzzles

1. Art of diagnosis and treatment of psychiatric disorders;
2. Stories of patients with psychiatric disorders; 3. Case histories of patients;
4. Mental Disorders; 5. Psychopharmacology; 6. Psychotherapy;
7. Contemporary practice of psychiatry; 8. Private practice of psychiatry; 9. Psychiatrists, physicians and therapists;

SOLVING PSYCHIATRIC PUZZLES

Table of Contents

SECTION THREE : APPENDICES

A human being is a part of the whole,
called by us "universe," a part limited
in time and space. He experiences himself,
his thoughts and feelings, as something separate
from the rest – a kind of optical delusion of his
consciousness. This delusion is a kind of prison for
us, restricting us to our personal decision and to affection
for a few persons nearest to us. Our task must be to free ourselves
from this prison by widening our circle of compassion to embrace all
living creatures and the whole nature in its beauty.

Albert Einstein

Weeping may linger for the night, but joy comes with the morning.

The Bible
Psalms

Divinity, lead me from the unreal to the real
From darkness into light
From death to immortality
Om peace peace peace

Upanishads

All that we are is the result of what we have thought. We are made of our thoughts; we are molded by our thoughts.

Buddha

Hope enables us to endure the hardships of life with courage and contentment. It emboldens us to encounter difficulties and overcome difficulties.

Zarathushtra (founder of Zoroastrianism)

We also boast in our sufferings, knowing that suffering produces endurance, and endurance produces character, and character produces hope, and hope does not disappoint . . .

The New Testament
Romans

He who has health has hope; and he who has hope has everything.

Muslim Proverb

This book is dedicated to my late parents, Dewan Chand Sethi and Ram Rakhi Wadhwa-Sethi; my late sister-in-law, Vimla Sethi; my brothers, Ram, Om and Suraj; my sister Kailash; my children Preeti, Deepti and Becky; and Dolores for her unconditional love, support and encouragements; as well as to my patients and their families and therapists who taught me the art of psychiatry.

Acknowledgments

Since the start of my private practice of psychiatry, I have been fascinated by the process of how emotionally and psychiatrically impaired people get well with medications and psychotherapy in a relatively short period of time. Further, as an immigrant to the USA, I have been impressed with the life stories of patients and their families, in coping with these illnesses.

Coming from a strong science background, I have been raising questions about the "how" and "why" of the recovery process, with the result that I felt driven to write these stories. In this process, about five years ago, I took classes in creative writing of short stories at the local college.

When I told my patients about the project, they brought their personal and family stories, and I learned so much about them that I did not know. They also shared that by this process they were able to make peace with themselves and their family. Further, they were willing to talk to my collaborator, George Jacobs, who crafted some of these stories for the book.

The names and identifying information about the patients have been changed to preserve confidentiality. The essence of their message, however, has not been changed.

I am grateful to all my patients who supported me in this project, and from whom I have learned a lot about humanity, interdependence, love and sufferings. This has made me a better human being and a better psychiatrist.

I am thankful to George Jacobs for steering me in the right direction and teaching me patience, that not every thing has to be done today.

I liked Traci Quinn's promptness in editing, and giving me an honest opinion about the project. Thanks a lot for your help.

My wife, Dolores, deserves special thanks for her unconditional love, support and ongoing encouragements with this and other projects.

My children, Preeti and Deepti, went through a part of the manuscript and gave me a good feedback. This has certainly facilitated our mutual bonding and love.

Lastly, I am grateful to Robert Golden, MD, Charles Nemeroff, MD, and Ranga Krishnan, MD, the respective Chairs of the Departments of Psychiatry at the University of North Carolina, Chapel Hill, North Carolina, Emory University at Atlanta, Georgia, and Duke University, Durham, North Carolina, for reading a part of the manuscript and giving their feedback.

Preface

Throughout human history there have been wars for acquiring more power through land, trade, religion and political conversion and domination, as well as extinction of races and religions, thus leading to human suffering. Human genes for survival adapted to these adversities and continue to reproduce. At the basic family unit, there are happy moments of falling in love, marriages, raising children, being successful at a trade, celebrating birthdays and festivals, and just trying to forget the sufferings of the destruction of life, demolition of property by bulldozers, rapes, lootings, and killing of people for differences in color, race and religion. According to Gandhi, love always triumphs over hatred and war.

Besides the physical sufferings and deaths of millions of innocent people, what happens to the mental sufferings? Does our brain chemistry adapt to forget the pains of deaths and sufferings, or does it becomes more sensitized to tell these stories in poems, paintings, religious books or just by oral traditions from one generation to the next? We should have had more post-traumatic stress disorder from one generation to the next if it was genetically ingrained. Further, why do psychiatric genes of schizophrenia, bipolar disorder, depression or anxiety not die with wars, diseases and famines? Are they part of the survival genes that make us human?

The incidence of major psychiatric disorders through different parts of the world is similar, independent of religion, socioeconomic, racial or regional differences. The common thread in the human race is shaped by the feelings of love, hatred, sorrow and joy emanating out of human bonds in family and social structure. These feelings are very important in raising children and building family, society and nations. Therefore, depressive feelings over the break-up of relationships, loss of job or business, or death of loved ones are universal and possibly essential for the survival of the human race.

Among all clinicians, psychiatrists and therapists are in a unique position to see the unfolding of a life story of a person in the form of a movie, whereas other physicians see only one part – cardiologists see the heart, and gastroenterologists see the colon. I sincerely hope that the future generation of psychiatrists will continue to see the whole human being rather than focus on "depression", "schizophrenia" or "panic disorder."

The stories described in this book could be true of patients in India, China, Japan, Germany, France, Russia, Spain, Mexico or Australia. I sincerely hope that through these stories you have a better appreciation of mental illness and psychiatry. Further, if this book has helped you to feel less stigmatized about mental illness, I would feel fortunate to have my mission accomplished.

CHAPTER 1

Introduction: The Art of Listening

Happiness and sorrow, highs and lows, encounters and departures mark the passing of time, but one thing remains unchanged: the will to become a better and more complete human being.

American Psychiatric Association
Art Association

She is barely four feet tall. From the Guilin province in southeast China, she has deep-set eyes, a light blue blouse with two buttons showing under her darker jacket, a proud Mongol nose, and a face with a hundred beautiful lines aiming toward a whisper of a smile. Almost irritated, almost laughing, she evokes my sister. She is a favorite portrait because, like all decent art, she begs the important questions: what kind of hardships have been known, did they strengthen or shatter, has there been more joy than sorrow, was there a time when all was gained or lost? Most of all, the sheer weight of her presence demands the viewer to admit the irreducible dignity of what it means to be a human being.

I feel the same creative joy in photography as in my psychiatric practice; they both demand precision, creativity and, above all else, respect. It is a reverence for the other that has nothing to do with you. It is the attempt to capture the sorrow, joy and universality of the human spirit, in all its wonder, ugliness and beauty. Through my own struggles, I have found that art and science meet together in the awe of mystery, or else they are neither art nor science.

Like crafts and the fine arts, psychiatry can tell us much about who we are. Sadly, the universal mask we place between the world and ourselves hinders every creative endeavor. I grew up in the Punjab, was educated in India, Germany, Mexico and the United States. I am an American to the core, and take my photographic portraits mainly in Asia and the Far East. It is remarkable that every society asks the same casual question, "How are you doing?" to which almost every individual has adapted the learned universal response, "I am doing fine," "I am OK."

The purpose of this book is to show how the science of psychiatry peels away the masks we wear, so patient and physician can identify the underlying causes of pain and heal them. Psychiatrists essentially have two primary colors on their palette. The first is the art of listening. As there are no blood tests or CAT scans to clearly identify the vast majority of mental illnesses, listening remains the primary tool a psychiatrist has to diagnose an illness or disorder. It is also the best instrument we have to confirm or change diagnoses as well as access and adjust treatment.

The second primary color in the psychiatrist's palette is the increasingly complex spectrum of pharmaceuticals. The discovery of Prozac (fluoxetine) by D.T. Wong in 1974 and its general use in the late 1980s were true landmarks in the development of psychiatric medications, one that accelerated the discovery of numerous other psychotropic drugs. Yet, the most powerful prescription a psychiatrist can ever give to a patient is hope. Having seen the humbling and astounding power of hope to begin healing, it would be unprofessional negligence for me not to look into the eyes of each new patient on his initial visit and tell him, "Together, we can make you better." Despite the lingering stigma of psychiatry, and the qualms many have about taking medications for mental health, the fact is that at least 90 percent of all mental illness is treatable. Psychiatry begins with respect for the individual dignity of every patient and the knowledge that there is hope.

This book is for those who suffer from mental illness, their loved ones, mental health workers, and other physicians to better understand the art, practice, and nature of psychiatry. The format will be to listen to the voices of patients in their own words so the reader can hear their suffering, feel their recovery and healing, and understand their ongoing struggle with mental illness.

As I read my patients' stories, I was surprised to learn new things about each person, even though I had treated all of them for at least several years. This should have been common sense: the more we learn about ourselves, our parents, children, spouses, and closest friends, the greater their mystery becomes. No matter how well we know a person, we never know her whole story.

This is also a challenge, a cry from the field of fifteen years of practice, to claim that psychiatry requires a unique relationship between patient and physician for the best possible healing to occur. If a person breaks his leg, then has several orthopedic surgeons in a group supervising his recovery, it is likely he will receive the best care possible. However, psychiatry demands an extended, individual, professional relationship of trust and respect between the physician and patient.

The brain is the most complex organ in the body, and mental illness is affected by heredity, health, environment, stressors, and so many other variables that a patient must see the same psychiatrist, over a period of time, to receive the chance of optimal care. The demise of this individual, one-on-one psychiatric practice must be one of the major topics of discussion in American public health. If not, patient and physician will continually be reduced to replaceable, interchangeable cogs in the vast medical industry.

Does Every Person Have Dignity?

One of the basic questions of what it means to live and die and be a human being is, "Are we unique?" Is every person so irreplaceable that you and I must regard him or her with dignity, regardless of personal history or station in life? It remains an open question. Various cultures, religions, philosophies, branches of science, and medicine have given very different answers as they work out their beliefs and theories in the hard reality of everyday life. Hinduism and Buddhism do not highly value the individual; Christianity teaches that each person is created in God's image. Yet, devout Christians have utterly opposing views concerning abortion, capital punishment, euthanasia, just war, etc. Regardless of the group we are born into, or affiliate with, each of us must personally deal with this fundamental question.

The only way I can answer is by telling you my story.

My mother's family was Hindu, while father was a scholar in the Sikh scriptures. Both were hard working, honest, and deeply religious. While we celebrated festivals from each faith, my mother deliberately rejected the Hindu caste system whereby some individuals are seen as a little less than gods, while others are literally treated as and called untouchables.

My parents came from stable middle class merchants and landowners. My father wore European clothes with a white turban. Mother wore the Punjabi shalwar-kameez (the traditional Indian loose pants covered by a long-sleeved tunic) with a dupatta covering her head. My father was a college graduate, while mother, as most Indian women in her time, was afforded only a fourth-grade education. Despite their differences, they treated each other with utter respect and admiration.

I was the youngest of six children. My uncles were wealthy businessmen and had large homes and shops in Phularwan, a city now in Pakistan. My favorite uncle was Channon Shah Wadhwa, a man of culture and extravagance. Beautiful calligraphies of framed Persian and Urdu poems lined the walls of his living room. He would recite poetry as he handed us money to buy sodas and ice cream. There was always plenty of food, milk, and pure-homemade Ghee, a sumptuous clarified butter. Uncle Wadhwa also had a wandering eye for beautiful women and fine whisky, a combination that created an unbroken battle between him and my aunt.

It was a richly textured and wonderful childhood. My father went on long business trips throughout the country, and he would send us dried fruits, sweets, cakes and cookies. When he returned home, it was with trunks of clothes for the family. Despite our prosperity, my mother was extraordinarily hard-working. She would wake before dawn, take a quick bath with cold water, and then prepare the portable coal-fire hearth called an angethi. She mixed wheat flour with water, kneading dough with both hands for chapatties and paranthas. Vegetables, garlic, ginger and tomatoes were cut to make subzies for breakfast, which we ate with homemade yogurt and hot tea or warm milk.

As there were no refrigerators, all the food had to be fresh, which meant going to the vegetable market and shops in the late afternoon.

After we left for school with a packed lunch, mother would wash our clothes with soap and water warmed in pans on the angethi. The laundry was beaten with a round bat, rinsed, and hand-wrung to dry in the sun. Then there were floors to be swept and a house to be cleaned for the visitors my father would bring home for lunch.

She would sit in the afternoon sun and take a brief rest, reading from her sacred scriptures, plying a spinning wheel to make thread, knitting sweaters, mending clothes, sometimes making us new clothes.

When we returned from school, we ate morning leftovers along with seasonal fruits, boiled milk with a thick crust, sometimes freshly made pikoras and sweets from the market. The routine would start all over again for the evening dinner. Though she could afford outside help, she never liked the idea of servants, and would rather do everything in her own way. She considered every person to be equal. There was no caste system in her personal faith or in her family. Without father knowing, she would kindly slip my sisters-in-law money to help their families. She never wore makeup, but always wore luminous, clean clothes. She was small, no more than five feet tall, thin, and braided her beautiful long white hair under the dupatta.

Our family continued to prosper, and we moved into a big house on Har Govind Street in Lahore, Punjab, where father also conducted his business. We had electricity and running water —life was good.

Everything changed in the summer of 1947, as I saw our neighbor's home burn to the ground. That summer we stood on our roof and watched houses and shops burning for miles.

Soon guns, swords, and weapons were hidden in the chimney. The military police came to our home at night to look for my brothers, who were fighting with local Hindu militia. So each night they stayed with a different friend or relative. My father and brother went to Delhi to look for a new home. When they returned in two weeks, we packed and sent what we could by train. We were in the middle of the greatest tragedy our land ever knew, as the British divided the subcontinent between Pakistan and India. Millions of Muslems were moved to Pakistan as Hindus, Sikhs, and those of other religions were also forced from their ancestral homes. We had lived together peaceably for centuries. Today, generations after the partition, there are still wars and hatred between the two nations, causing such senseless poverty and exploitation for the poorest of the poor.

We arrived in Delhi unharmed, but millions were looted, raped, murdered, separated forever from their families, losing property and every belonging. It was a time of despair as many parents committed suicide when they could no longer take care of their families.

My father tried to establish his business from almost nothing. In September of the year we moved to Delhi, the Yamuna River flooded, and our house was covered by five feet of water. We took refuge in our home along with the wild animals, snakes, rats and dogs that swam in, also clinging to life. As the youngest, I was with my mother the entire time. I shall always remember the evening when there was no food and I went with her as she asked for food from strangers. The great American writer William Faulkner wrote, "Aye, grief fades, we know that, but try to ask the tear ducts if they have forgotten how to weep." I still cry — never forgetting, always remembering that evening in a wasteland of fear and death.

I tried to ignore my world at home and focused all my energy toward school. I passed my pre-university exams with distinction, and went to a prestigious Banaras Hindu University 400 miles away to study Pharmacy. I wanted my parents to visit, but poverty and poor health kept us apart. After completing my master's degree, I received a scholarship to study in Germany. Traveling the cities of Eastern and Western Europe, I wished my parents could come and see the marvels of those lands. However, after leaving India, I never saw my mother again. She died a few weeks prior to my returning to India.

Whenever I go to a Hindu Temple or Sikh Gurudwara, the women still sit on one side and the men on the other, I look among the women for the image of my mother with her long white braided hair, soft smile, and complete humility. The images of the women are familiar, but I leave sad and diminished.

My Unitarian Universalist Church of Charlotte in North Carolina has a memorial garden where I placed my parents' names. There is solace when I am there. I stand before them in silence, touch the plates, place a flower or leaf, light incense or a candle, and I remember their story.

So, I take pictures, searching for joy, sorrow, and beauty, but in most of my pictures I am trying to grasp the universality of the human spirit. You can see it in their faces, dignity born of moving on despite it all, never giving up, and forever continuing the story.

Our question comes home, "Are human beings unique? Must we regard every person with dignity regardless of what they have done or been?" When I sit in front of a patient who has been in and out of psychiatric hospitals, or one who has been lying to clinicians and wandered from psychiatrist to psychiatrist, must I give these persons dignity and respect? Do I listen? I could not touch my parents' names, or tell their story, if I did not.

As a biomedical scientist with over 80 publications in my first professional life, I asked questions and solved the mysteries with experimental bench research. My office is my lab now; I try to solve the psychiatric puzzle of each patient with the same zeal and fervor as I used to do with my experiments in the lab.

How Does a Psychiatrist Listen?

Sixty to seventy percent of those who walk in my office are referred by their therapists, mental health counselors, or primary care physicians. Current and former patients refer another twenty percent. Increasingly, people are finding their psychiatrists through lists provided by their in-network managed health care groups. Of these, many simply call two or three names and schedule an appointment with the one who can see them the earliest.

During their initial visit, patients have 45 to 50 minutes or so with their psychiatrist. Like many others, when I began my practice I asked patients to fill out long forms that might ramble on for fifty questions. I gave these up. The reason is that I found myself looking at the form instead of the person. Like a good family doctor, a psychiatrist can eliminate or have a feeling for numerous illnesses just by looking at a patient. Even how a person dresses can give important signals to what is going on in his or her life. Is there trembling or shaking, can they focus, is the person able to look at you? All these are critical signs. So now, I look and write as they talk.

When you go to a primary care physician, a nurse often measures your weight and blood pressure before you see the doctor. In the same way, the first thing I do is ask the patient to step on the scale. While this may seem odd at first ("Isn't he supposed to be trying to figure out what is going on in my head?"), weight factors are important. Weight may indicate an eating disorder; it may also affect potential prescriptions. It is also important to have a baseline for subsequent visits to see if there are side effects of a medication, causing weight gain or loss.

Then, I ask the basic questions of age, marital status, and occupation. They are not simply data for insurance forms. If a person is single, it generally means he is self-supporting and statistically has a smaller support system than those who are married. There are also age-specific mental illnesses or disorders. Depression among the elderly is a relatively common illness often dismissed as a "natural" part of growing old or dementia. There are a number of mental illnesses triggered at different stages in life, particularly in adolescence, young adulthood, and menopause.

In the United States, we are defined by what we do, so how a person is functioning in her career suggest tremendous stressors that may trigger certain illnesses. In addition, of course, mental illness often changes or threatens a person's ability not only to work, but in all areas of functioning.

All psychiatric symptoms can be broken down into two categories—qualitative and quantitative. Qualitative symptoms, unique to the schizophrenia spectrum of disorders, are hearing voices, seeing things, and having paranoia or delusions.

Most other symptoms in psychiatry are quantitatively different from the normal, which could vary from culture to culture. This is where one has to listen to the patient, as the essential question becomes: "Is this symptom in a normal range for this person?" A manic episode may indicate a bipolar disorder, but the symptom may be closer to an explosive temper or minor mood swing, which is not a manic stage. You have to listen, because you do not want to go down the wrong diagnostic road too soon. After the top blanks are filled in, my next question is, "Tell me what's going on?" This is when you literally listen to the rate of a person's voice. A person's speed of speaking usually reflects his rate of thinking. This is something we all know on a daily basis. If someone is speaking very slowly, or if his or her speech is halting or broken, you sense a vagueness of thought or inability to focus. *What* they are thinking about is a different matter.

Normally, patients are quite honest, and they become more honest with subsequent visits. It is against human nature to tell everything about yourself the first time you meet someone, even a psychiatrist. The question, "Is there anything else I need to know that I have not asked or you would like to share with me?" may be answered on subsequent visits, especially when there has been physical and sexual abuse. Again, this is another reason why there must be a one-on-one relationship between the patient and psychiatrist. Trust takes time, and it only grows in mutual respect. Therefore, people must be given total respect as unique individuals. Yes, they may still mislead you, but they may also tell you the truth and grow closer to healing with each visit.

As a person begins to speak, you need to hear the spaces between words and ask specific questions that may be affecting the presenting symptoms. They may have had previous episodes of depression, panic attacks, or are particularly stressed, while some patients suffer symptoms for no apparent reason. Histories of hospitalization and suicide attempts need to be known so as to assess the severity of illness. Likewise, any suicidal or homicidal thoughts with any plans and intent must be investigated. If there is any potential for suicide, the person's safety immediately becomes more crucial than his or her privacy.When a person has actually spent some time thinking the world would be better off without him, I immediately call a spouse, close friend, even an employer if there is no one else. We all talk together on a speakerphone. The more open you are with a patient, the better. If a person has suicidal thoughts that are not serious enough to require hospitalization, I ask the friend or spouse to take any guns or potentially dangerous medications out of the home, and be with the patient until the crisis is over.

As patients are describing their symptoms, I try to put them into different diagnostic categories, and explore further the extent and durations of them. Also, I want to know which are more recent and which have been going on for a longer time or even their whole life. It is important to know the medical history and alcohol, nicotine, caffeine, or other substance abuse history, and history of current and past medications, as well as over–the-counter medications. In addition, what medications have been tried for their psychiatric conditions, did they have any side effects, and at what dosages? Patients are unique in their need for psychiatric medications. They must be titrated (slowly adding specific amounts) individually without any side effects. The dosages recommended by the drug companies have been determined on severely ill patients in a university or medical research setting for only one psychiatric disorder. In a community or outpatient office setting, we see patients with two or three psychiatric diagnoses, and thus our choice of medications and dosages are generally different. Further, as we have more choices of medications with different mechanisms of actions, we are successfully using combinations of medications to alleviate symptoms.

As people tell their stories, family histories are critically important. The ages and names of siblings are recorded, along with their profession and where they are living. It tells me a lot. Biological brothers and sisters have a similar genetic makeup. If a patient says a parent, uncle, aunt, or even a grandparent suffered from mental illness or was drinking heavily, it gives a significant insight. It is also helpful to know the age and name of the spouse and the general family constellation, not descriptive to the last detail, but with enough information to get a clear picture. There will always be a debate between the effects of nature versus nurture among professionals. The important issue is that when a psychiatrist listens to a patient, all factors must be considered. Therefore, I also ask about current stressors, such as job loss, bad relationships, marital conflicts, physical illness, moving, financial aspects, deaths and grieving, and try to determine what influence they have on the symptoms. I also ask about their eating habits, exercise, and sleep patterns. I want to know their functioning at work, school, home, and social setting on a scale of one to ten. Likewise, I record the severity of symptoms of depression, panic attacks, anxiety, paranoia, obsessive compulsiveness, tempers, mood swings, etc., on a scale of one to ten. If there are relationship issues, I ask them to rate their impairment on the same scale.

In a brief social and developmental history I want to know where they were born and raised, and if there were any physical, emotional, or sexual traumas while growing up. How was the relationship of their parents with each other, and what kind of work did they do? In addition, how far did the patient go to school, at what age was he or she married, and how many children do they have? If there is more than one marriage, I ask about reasons for divorce. Also what kind of work they do, how long they have been in this city, and what kind of support (church, family, friends, AA members, coworkers) they have?

In a Mental Status Examination, I record their appearance, dress, grooming, cooperation, eye contact, anxiousness, mood, memory, intelligence, insight, judgment, speech, thought process, feelings of paranoia, delusions or hallucinations, alertness, if they are in or out of touch with reality, and any oddness of behavior, or hostility.

Before giving the patient my impression of what is going on, I always ask if there is anything that I have not asked, or anything else the patient would like to share with me that is important.

Further, if they have come with a spouse or parent, would they mind if I talk to them as well, and is there anything that I must not tell them? In most cases, I give the patient (in the presence of the accompanying person), a summary of my findings and ask them if there is anything that they wish to add or modify.

With these data in hand, I summarize my findings, and give them my impression of their diagnosis, and discuss different treatment possibilities, including medications and therapy. I also give a rationale for my choices of medications and their side effects. If there are no questions, I give them a return appointment within 10 to 15 days.

All psychiatric diagnoses have three different levels of severity — mild, moderate, and severe. Milder forms of psychiatric symptoms can be successfully treated with psychotherapy or counseling. There are data in the literature that similar changes in brain functioning are produced from medication or psychotherapy. Further research data are very convincing that in moderate to severe psychiatric conditions, a combination therapy of medications and psychotherapy are superior to either.

A formal psychiatric diagnosis is described in five parts: Axis I to V. Axis I describes the psychiatric diagnoses such as Major Depressive Disorder, Schizophrenia, Bipolar Affective Disorder, Panic Disorder, Anxiety Disorder, Bulemia, Obsessive Compulsive Disorder, Substance or Alcohol Abuse/Dependence, Dementia, Attention Deficit Disorder, etc. Axis II describes Personality Disorders and Mental Retardation. There are ten Personality Disorders described in the current diagnostic manual of mental illnesses, such as Paranoid, Dependent, Antisocial, Narcissistic, Avoidant, Borderline, Histrionic, Schizoid etc. I avoid diagnosing anyone with Personality Disorder, as there is an overlap of symptoms between Axis I and Axis II, and we do not fully understand the relationship of Axis I symptoms with Axis II. There is also serious continuing debate among the scientific community about the validity of Axis II disorders. Axis III describes general medical conditions, such as hypertension, coronary artery disease, arthritis, fibromyalgia, stroke, etc. Axis IV describes psycho-social and environmental problems, such as job, housing, relationship, financial, etc. Axis V describes the Global Assessment of Functioning (GAF) Scale from ten to 100 — ten being the worst and 100 being the best.

Due to the overlapping nature of psychiatric symptoms, it is very important to keep in mind the hierarchy of psychiatric diagnoses. At the top are the medical conditions and prescriptions, including over-the-counter medications. For example, if someone is taking a medication that contains caffeine, ephedrine, or stimulants to reduce weight or be more alert, a psychiatrist has to be careful not to diagnose symptoms as an anxiety disorder when the symptoms may be side effects from these or other medications. Further, if there is a hypo- or hyperthyroid condition, it can mimic psychiatric symptoms, and thus must be corrected first. Next in the hierarchy is abuse of alcohol, caffeine, nicotine, or other substances. One has to be certain symptoms are not the result of withdrawal, abuse, or dependence on these substances. Next on this ladder, in descending order, are Schizophrenia and other Psychotic Disorders, Dementia, Mood Disorders (Bipolar Disorder,

Depression), Anxiety Disorders (Panic Disorder, Social Phobias, Obsessive-Compulsive Disorder), Impulse Control Disorders, Adjustment Disorders, Attention Deficit Disorder, and Personality Disorder. I explain this hierarchy to my patients so they have a better understanding of their diagnosis.

In the follow-up appointment of 15 to 20 minutes, I examine any improvement or deterioration of symptoms, including any side effects from medications. In addition, is there any change in the person's functioning? At this point, further changes in medications and dosages are made and explained to the patient. This process continues until the symptoms are abated. The progress of psychotherapy, if any, is also noted.

For various reasons, a person rarely visits a psychiatrist until the pain or fallout of symptoms becomes serious. Thus, 80 to 90 percent of those who make an initial appointment can be helped by medications and psychotherapy. The far greater danger is in avoiding treatment. There are still lingering stigmas in our culture that keep people from seeking help.

Here are a few of the most common:

- **Assumption**: Psychiatry is an inexact science and relatively new branch of medicine.

  Fact: Psychiatry is the oldest branch of medicine. Founded in 1844, the *American Journal of Psychiatry* is the oldest continuously published medical specialty journal in the United States. Since the publication of DSM III in 1980, and DSM IV in 1994, and discovery of new medications, psychiatry is becoming a better clinical science, equivalent to other clinical disciplines of medicine.

- **Assumption**: Taking drugs for mental illness is a sign of moral or emotional weakness and is different from taking prescriptions for "physical illnesses."

  Fact: Mental illness is a physical illness. Just as all organs are affected by a combination of genetics, environmental factors, and structural/chemical imbalances, so too is the brain. The brain is the most complex physical organ in the human body.

- **Assumption**: Pharmaceuticals prescribed by a psychiatrist are foreign (thus potentially harmful) to the body and the brain's activity.

  Fact: Every type of food we eat is composed of chemicals. The brain is a wonderfully intricate organ that uses chemicals and electrical charges to transmit information and preserve its own health. Most medications enable the brain to restore its natural chemical balance.

- **Assumption**: Mental illness is not treatable, or does not improve without years of exhaustive treatment.

  Fact: Ninety percent of all mental illness is treatable within weeks to a few months of diagnosis. "There is hope -- together we can make you better!"

A Very Brief History of Psychiatry

It is understandable why people are often confused about the differences between psychologists and psychiatrists. Many pioneers of psychological theory were physicians who created hypotheses of human development, trying to answer such questions as: "What environmental stressors injure the mind?" "At what stages of life do these occur?" "What is universal in the ways we think, feel, and develop?" and "What are the best methods to heal mental illness?"

Of course, the best known of these physicians was Sigmund Freud, who published his most important work, *The Ego and the Id,* in 1923. This seminal work was the culmination of decades of Freud's observations with his patients in Vienna; it elaborated the first system of psychoanalytic psychology. One of the most important theories of Freudian analysis was the presence of the "unconscious," referring to the part of the mind that is inaccessible to the conscious mind and can only be reached through psychoanalytical techniques.

Several of Freud's early supporters had reservations to his psychoanalytical theories that our personality is formed through psychosexual developmental phases. Two of these set up their own "schools of thought" concerning the mind and its development. Alfred Adler developed the theory of individual psychology and Carl Jung broke with Freud and is known as the founder of analytical psychology. It is important to understand that this great flowering of psychological theories in the early twentieth century was generally separate from those who were researching the biochemical and physiological properties of the human brain.

American psychiatry was founded two generations before Freud, when the superintendents of 13 mental health hospitals met in Philadelphia to form the Association of Medical Superintendents of the American Institutions for the Insane, thankfully abbreviated to the AMSAII. Soon after they met, in 1844, they published the first edition of the *American Journal of Insanity* and began collecting data on the statistics of idiotsy (insanity). This journal would become the *American Journal of Psychiatry.*

Benjamin Rush, a signer of the Declaration of Independence, was an attending physician at the Pennsylvania General Hospital. Rush is often referred to as the father of American psychiatry because of his work, *Medical Inquiries and Observations upon the Diseases of the Mind.*Rush outlined the treatment of mental illness, which included physical measures such as bloodletting, starvation, purgatives, and leeches, as well as psychological (behavioral) techniques of: memorization, music therapy, shaming, fear, pain, and terror.

Dr. Thomas Kirkbride was the first to introduce treatments that were more humane, abolishing strait-jackets and discouraging terms such as "asylum" and "madhouse."

By 1881, six diagnoses of mental illnesses were described: mania, melancholia, monomania, dementia, dipsomania, and epilepsy. The next year Osler's *Principles and Practice of Medicine* added hysteria, alcoholism, morphine addiction, and obesity.

Scientists and physicians began to bring relative order to psychiatric diagnosis in the beginning of the twentieth century. There were also important advances in studying the physical properties of brain diseases. Emil Kraeplin in Germany differentiated schizophrenia from manic-depressive psychosis. In addition, Alzheimer, Nissel, and Broadmann were making significant contributions to the description and diagnosis of brain disorders.

Noguchi and Moore demonstrated *T. pallidum* as the cause of neurosyphilis in 1913. Four years later, the first biological psychiatric research facility was founded in Munich, Germany, under the leadership of Kraeplin. It is interesting to note that Freud was dealing with patients who were in an office setting whereas Kraeplin was collecting clinical data on severely ill hospital patients.

In 1950, the World Health Organization published Volume 6 of the International Classification of Diseases (ICD-6). This work served as the basis for APA's first *Diagnostic and Statistical Manual of Mental Disorders* (DSM-1). The ICD was updated in 1952 and 1968, bringing some order to the discipline, but even the 1968 edition only listed the names of mental disorders.

Whenever there is a rapid development of a science or technology, there is a lag time before international standards are created. The establishment of standard time zones did not occur until the advent of trains and people had to know arrival and departure times. Before then, the time was whatever the town church or courthouse clock said it was. Something had to be done as trains began to run between cities with various times. The same is somewhat true in the current development of computers, whose programmers are still working on standard operating systems, or at least ones that can communicate with each other.The same was true of psychiatry. There was no standardization of psychiatric terminology and diagnostic criteria until DSM-III was published in 1980 along with its revisions in 1987 (DSM IIIR) and 1994 (DSM IV). These publications gave, for the first time, specific diagnostic criteria for the description of mental disorders throughout the country and the world. It meant there was uniform nomenclature, and psychiatrists were able to communicate using the same language and meaning for various psychiatric conditions.

Throughout the twentieth century, a growing distinction developed between those who were diagnosing and treating mental illness through the psychological theories of Freud, Jung, Adler, Skinner, Rogers, and other researchers who were specifically concerned with the biochemical causes and treatments of mental illness with medications. This became the distinction between psychology and psychiatry.

Today, psychologists and psychotherapists have various educational backgrounds including: master's degrees in social work, psychology, divinity, as well as doctorate degrees in psychology. Despite these educational differences, national accrediation associations and state licencing boards have standardized test requirements. These therapists base their clinical work on a variety of psychological schools in treating mental conditions through various non-pharmaceutical methods.

Psychiatrists are those individuals who have earned a medical degree (MD) and are practicing physicians who have specialized their medical practice through a four- to five-year hospital-based residency program in psychiatry. Psychiatrists treat patients both in hospital and office settings. Generally, psychiatrists specialize in child and adolescent, adult and/or geriatric psychiatry. They diagnose and treat psychiatric disorders with the help of pharmaceuticals and psychotherapy.

Before 1950, the only biological treatment for severe mental illness was electroshock or electroconvulsive therapy (ECT).Without other medications, many patients' symptoms were so severe that long-term hospitalization was the only choice. Eventually, over half a million patients were in state mental hospitals (not including private facilities) in the United States.

The discovery of chlorpromazine (Thorazine), and its successful treatment of schizophrenia, was a revolution in psychiatry. Thankfully, it brought healing and spurred the development of other antipsychotic medications. Patients were able to leave state hospitals and receive care at outpatient community mental health centers.

Monoamine oxidase inhibitors were also developed in the late 1950s, which proved effective in treating depression. Numerous symptoms of depression are caused by the overly rapid absorption of naturally produced chemicals in the brain. MAO inhibitors cause the breakdown of neurotransmitter amines and other amino compounds in the body to slow down, and thereby increase the levels of these chemicals in the brain and body. Like all medications, the most successful in treating mental illness are those that help the body return to its natural chemical balance. These MAO inhibitors, however, had negative interactions with many foods. The severe limitations they placed on patient's diets reduced their popularity.

By the late 1950s, drugs were synthesized with similar chemical structures to chlorpromazine; imipramine was one of the more successful of these medications in treating depression.

Before 1950, barbiturates were widely used to treat anxiety and insomnia. They were effective but had a narrow range between their therapeutic and toxic dosages. A relative increase in the prescribed use triggered an overdose. The sheer availability of barbiturates in a prescription bottle was dangerous for patients who were potentially suicidal. Benzodiazepines discovered in the 1960s were much safer and are still used to treat anxiety, panic disorder and insomnia. The use of lithium salt in alleviating symptoms of mania was discovered in the 1970s and was another milestone in the development of biological psychiatry. Safer and more effective medications have been developed in the past 30 years. A description of these and other medications are included in the Appendix.

Of the top ten causes of disability in the world, four are mental illnesses. Depression is the leading cause of disability, followed by tuberculosis, traffic accidents, alcohol use, self-inflicted injuries, manic-depressive illness, war, violence, schizophrenia, and iron deficiency anemia. Additionally, for patients who have medical and psychiatric illnesses, the medical conditions do not improve unless the psychiatric conditions are treated.

Because of these advances, psychiatry is becoming a clinical science, but like all medicine, it will always remain an art and a craft. Ultimately, it can only be understood in the doing of it, as the puzzles of the human mind are unraveled. I invite you along on this journey as we listen to the voices of patients in their own words, and go through other assorted stories. Welcome to the journey.

Milestones in Physiological and Medical Psychiatry

- •1866 — George Mendel discovers the principles of heredity
- •1895 — Roentgen invents the X-ray
- •1906 — Golgi and Raunly Cajal win the Nobel Prize for discovering synapses in the brain.
- •1910 — Tomas Moran discovers chromosomes
- •1917 — Wagner-Jauregg wins the Nobel Prize for the treatment of syphilis by malaria toxins.
- •1921 — Loewi discovers the first neurotransmitter — acetylcholine
- •1929 — Berger invents the EEG
- •1935 — Moniz performs the fist lobotomy
- •1938 — The first electroshock treatment
- •1949 — John Cade discovers the beneficial effects of lithium
- •1952 — Laborit discovers the first antipsychotic drug—

chlorpromazine (Thorazine)

- 1953 — Watson and Crick discover the structure of the DNA molecule
- 1963 — Sternbach with Roche Labs discover the drug diazepam (Valium)
- 1973 — Snyder and Pert discover endorphin
- 1974 — D. T. Wong discovers fluoxetin (Prozac)
- 1972 — Housfield invents the CAT scan
- 1981 — The PET scan is invented
- 2000 — Working drafts of the human genome are completed

SECTION ONE :

VOICES OF PATIENTS

CHAPTER 2

I Am Grateful

Whate'er its mission, the soft breeze can come
To none more grateful than to me; escaped
From the vast city, where I long had pined
A discontented sojourner, now free,
Free as a bird to settle where I will.

William Wordsworth

Memories are strange; the ones that really matter are small, little things. It is the gluey, slippery smell of fresh mimeographed paper that frames my childhood at Steel Elementary — an old, three-story, brick-on-brick building. You could see the black steel fire escape from every side. On the inside, the school was a warm place with many friends; I did well. The teachers liked me, and I earned good grades. Until Mrs. Markawitz said, "Your handwriting is a mess; my son is in kindergarten, and he can write better than you can."

A math teacher of all things, she was well-dressed, stout, and looked past middle age from eyes that were not in the third grade. I did well in her class, but with every missed question she watched and named me "scatterbrain." The name stuck; children smell blood keener than sharks.

The three of us lived in a tiny two-bedroom house in Baldwin, Long Island. The house itself was an island in an upper middle-class town of 35,000. I always wanted brothers and sisters.

However, Mom said she "did not want to go through that." There was a brief season when she went to St. Joseph's to talk to the Father about adoption. For some reason it never went any further than talking.

Mom was two years older than Dad. The main thing she believed in was keeping secrets. She eternally claimed to be two years younger than she was. When I was in my 30s and Mom in her 60s, by chance I found her birth certificate. She said, "Oh, they must have made a mistake." Her story never changed.

There were so many things you just couldn't talk about in my house.

Dad was a handsome man with thick, dark, curly hair. Four and a half packs of Winston's a day kept him thin as a curve. He showed little emotion, few hugs, but I felt a sincere love from him. It came through actions. With a faint smile but an intense caring, he handed me change from his pocket. I loved all kinds of candy, but whenever Dad gave me money, I would buy some kind of chocolate, always chocolate, flat Hershey bars, sometimes with almonds, Snickers and Milky Ways. In high school, Dad knew I wanted a tan leather coat with long fringes for my birthday. All the cool kids looked like urban Indians. It must have cost him a week's salary.

One afternoon, my neighbor Carol and I were sitting in her back yard, when for some reason, I told her my real name, "Betsy, Betsy Lieberman."

Mom called me in the house, and with eyes I could not question said, "There are some things we just don't talk about."

I knew the details. Dad was born Herbert Lieberman, the youngest of six children. Dad became a Linden when his brother's wife wanted the family to change their name before she married.

Five of the children were able to leave Germany. Jerry, Gerhard and Ruth were sent to America through a program called "A Thousand Children," where young Jews were sponsored by American families before the war. Aunt Ellie ended up in the Dominican Republic. The youngest girl, Edith, was never heard from again. My father was the last child to leave. My grandfather spent some time in a concentration camp, but was released because of his status as a decorated WWI veteran.

Omma and Oppa moved to New York. When they were at our house, another level of stillness pressed down around us. Oppa never raised his voice, "in case the neighbors might hear." With so many others from the same place and generation, my grandparents followed the diaspora to Miami Beach to be among friends.

Mom was Catholic, and I think she believed. Yet, there was a greater deference for my neutrality, so neither practiced their religion. If I have to label myself in those terms, I am a Humanist and have always felt comfortable believing this life is all there is.

Somehow, I had become fashionable again by junior high; most of the kids didn't know my past. Part of it is that I have always been able to begin a conversation. Even in the dark times, I could — and needed — to talk to anyone. By high school, I was street-wise, boy-smart, and pretty. It didn't hurt that Lonnie walked me home every afternoon. Lonnie was the cool, bad guy, who all the girls wanted; for some reason, he paid attention to me every day in school.

But popularity has its embarrassing side.

My mother's phobias had seemed benign at first: flying, claustrophobia, heights, loud noises – firecrackers were the worst; the Fourth of July was a bad day. Her fears were like the little skin tags on her neck, just something weird or gross that came along with being a parent. I never thought anything was seriously wrong. Then she began to complain that the things she watched on television did not make sense. One commercial showed a tissue in the wind. *"That's not real. They are just making it up. It's not real."* She kept saying everything was *"crazy"* as she questioned my father and me, *"Why are they doing these things?"*

It was frightening, and I did not want to be around her. Once, she came home unexpectedly. I hid with my friend in the basement, making up some story until we could slip out of the house without being seen. It just wasn't cool having a crazy mother.

Once we were at my grandparents' and I heard Dad say, *"It is happening again."*

Again? This had happened before? When? Why didn't anyone tell me? I felt betrayed, deceived; I never knew there was another time. Looking back, I understand why Dad didn't want, or need, to place that burden on me, but I felt lied to at the time.

There were so many taboos. The house rule became, "Do not upset Mom, or she may have another nervous breakdown." Yet there was always another anyway, two or three a year when she would be away for a month a longer. A neighbor took me to see her; these visits were very short, and I always felt uncomfortable. There must have been many trips to the hospital, but only one is clear in my memory. She had just received an electroshock therapy treatment. When we walked out of the hospital, I remember thinking she looked like a zombie — there was nothing in her eyes, not even any secrets.

When she was home, her illness focused on the television, once again. *"That's not real, Thing's are not right. It's not real . . ."*

As things got worse, she was afraid to be by herself. One day after school, she became so stressed she kept saying, "You need to call your father," until finally she threw the phone at me.

Was it my fault?

I was scared and guilty; I didn't think Mom would ever be normal again. And there was a darker thought haunting those years: Would I grow up to have *"The Problem"*? Mom and I didn't look or act alike. It spooked me when a boyfriend once said, "If there were a roomful of mothers and daughters, anyone could tell you belonged together."

But there had been signs. When I was a small child, I couldn't handle any kind of change. I remember when my parents changed the wallpaper in the living room. I was so upset they had to finish their work while I slept that night. Once, I spilled a cup of tea and the teabag clung to my leg. Mom and Dad took me to the doctor, who tried to put some purple salve on the burn. I kept thinking, then began screaming, "It doesn't belong there; this isn't right; my leg is not supposed to look like that." A few years later, I started crying in front of a neighbor while my parents were putting new siding on the house. Only our neighbor asked what was wrong.

In high school, I smoked grass to fit in, but it made me feel paranoid. Not the normal teenage fear of getting into trouble, but the feeling that events were oddly connected to me. *"The light just shut off -- is it me? Does it have something to do with me?"* It wasn't guilt; it was something worse. It was the same paranoia I saw in my mother: *"Things are not right; is it my fault?"* There was always a fretfulness hovering about, stealing the moment out of living.

That fretfulness still shows itself, following me in a nervous laugh that I have never been able to shake. It comes from a lack of confidence in what I am saying — a worried giggle to break the ice. Even though I have always been extroverted, the first person to talk on the bus or elevator, the laugh comes when I don't know what to say or when I can't let others in.

After high school, I took a few classes at the local community college. I was smart enough for a university, but it was something my parents neither expected nor encouraged. I went to work, and I did well. I started with Liberty Mutual in Manhattan as a file clerk and soon moved up to being a statistical coder. I was afraid to leave home for several years; the commute was only an hour on the train and the subway.

Computers were just starting to be used in offices, and their language came easy for me. I bought a condo in Rockland County. The commute was an hour and a half if everything went perfectly, but usually two. It began with a drive to Fort Lee, New Jersey, then a bus from one side of the George Washington

Bridge to the other. Then I took the A Train from 168th all the way through Manhattan to Fulton Street, where there was a stop in the building.

There was a lot of traveling, as I taught other insurance people how to use computers. In 1985, I moved to Charlotte, North Carolina, with friends from the company. At first, things were good — exciting. I was working with quality assurance, making good money, which went a lot further without the commute expenses and high rents.

I had a lot of friends and was never without a date, but I was in my mid-twenties before any relationships lasted more than a few weeks. The guys I dated could sense I was nervous, and it must have made them uncomfortable.

Things got better. After a couple of long-term relationships, I became more at ease with myself around men. But then my friends began to marry, and for the first time in my life, I found myself alone and lonely. Then came the anxiety. Sleeping was hard. So many nights passed with little or no sleep at all. I remember moving from the bedroom to the couch each night, hoping a change in position would help. The night passed slowly; the sound of defeat came every night at 3 a.m., when the police car drove through the neighborhood.

Things began to fall apart. I was having trouble focusing. Soon, even simple tasks and decisions seemed impossible. What top should I wear? Which shoes? Soon every moment was frightening; I was so nervous that I couldn't stay alone.

My good friend Mary let me stay with her, but after a few weeks it became clear that my state of mind was getting worse. I was a burden on my friend and knew things were getting beyond her ability to take care of me.

For the first time in my life, I went to a psychiatrist and began counseling, but it wasn't helping. I realized I needed to be hospitalized. I felt safe and cared for at Cedar Springs Hospital. I didn't have to think about what to eat. But things weren't getting any better.

Kind people from my company worked with the doctors at the Charlotte hospital. It was decided I should be near my family in New York. I was so nervous, unable to make decisions; I was grateful they were being made for me.

When I checked in to Mercy Hospital, it had been twenty years since my mother's last hospitalization. With the stress of my illness, she became sick again. I felt incredibly guilty; I thought her illness was entirely my fault.

Mercy was anything but. The psychiatric wing was a sterile place, locked doors, just a regular hospital room with lots of worthless group therapy.

Therapists have never been very helpful for me. Most seemed like they were not interested in who the patients actually were — in their stories. There seemed to be as little structure to what they were doing as in the daily routine they constructed. There was one therapist in particular, a woman with long dark hair. Her therapy session was a lecture. The clearest point she made was, "I have to do this today; it is part of my agenda." She said there are four kinds of people — aggressive, passive, passive-aggressive, and one I can't remember. She labeled me passive-aggressive. The diagnosis was not distressing, but it did nothing to make things better. I couldn't make the correlation between the definition and my state of mind. The psychiatrists' tests were just as useless. There were no abnormalities in my abilities to reason, no cause for my problems. It was decided I should be admitted to a psychiatric hospital.

Jewish Hospital had a good reputation in the city, and I felt much more at ease there. It was a campus setting, and I made a lot of friends my age who seemed to care about me. They were kind, and my doctor showed me simple kindness and empathy. I trusted him. He actually cared about me as a real person: I was not a diagnosis or an illness to be charted.

I remember one of the girls sitting me down. She styled my hair and put on makeup. Everyone said, "You look so beautiful." It felt good to be fussed over.

My psychiatrist told me I should undergo electro-shock treatments (ECTs). The image of my mother when I was a teenager kept flashing through my mind. However, the treatments did help her despite the side effects, so I decided to proceed with it. After three to four treatments, my thoughts were clearer. It was a time of lightness; I was connected to the moment. I felt there was hope that I would get better. My doctor said I required eight treatments. With these, I suffered some short-term memory loss, but the names of people and places returned in a few weeks.

Shortly after the treatments, I was released from Jewish Hospital. I flew back to Charlotte and started back to work in a few days. Then, for the first time, the manic stage set in. Everything seemed fine -- in fact, I felt great, better than I ever felt in my life. The only little problem was that I thought the entire world was revolving around me — I thought I was doing spectacular work at the office and that my supervisors were going to promote me any day. I thought the people at the radio stations knew what I was doing every moment, because they were playing songs just for me, sometimes sending messages that only I could understand. Once I found a cassette tape that I thought someone left for me to lead me in the right direction.

Naturally, my friends and co-workers found this behavior a bit more frightening than my previous anxiety and depression. Even though they tried to be supportive, they began to distance themselves. At the time, I could not understand why they were leaving me alone and backing away. It was incredibly painful.

There was one person who listened. John did not back away. It is easy to cross inappropriate boundaries, especially when men and women confide in and help each other. It is especially risky when someone is as vulnerable as I was. Thankfully, John knew where the lines were as he gently helped me to see my behavior was not rational and that I needed help. He was not spooked by the parts of my illness that scared others. My psychiatrist prescribed a medication that balanced my moods, and for a while, life became stable.

When I returned to work this time, attitudes were different. I was told my former supervisory position would be too stressful. I enjoyed the new work, came to terms with the decision, and slowly began to regain respect from my co-workers. It is amazing how closely our mental health is connected to how well we are doing in our careers.

Life was relatively stable for two years until my position with the company changed. Departments were restructured, and for the first time in my life, I found myself responsible for assignments for which I had neither the proper training nor the skills. I was left searching for what I was supposed to be doing until I received an unsatisfactory evaluation and was placed on probation. It was hard, because work was the one place where I had always done well, a place where I met goals and found stability.

I was assigned to a data entry position. I hated my job but was afraid to try anything else. Most of all, I was terrified of failing. My social life was also falling apart. I didn't have any close friends, and the guy I was dating was understanding but did not want any commitment — no obligations. I finally said goodbye.

The same anxiety symptoms returned: lack of sleep, an inability to focus or make the simplest decisions, and a completely helpless feeling that never went away. Each day was clouded with a frightening anxiety, as if I were in the middle of a difficult exam or speaking in front of a large group of people. Someone once said we can endure pain if we know it is going to end, or if we know it is going to go on forever, but what is unendurable is feeling such pain with only the faint hope that it might go away. I was losing up to a pound a day, and I had little to lose. I remember talking to my mother during this time and telling her, "The thing I am most terrified of is dying."

There were several more hospitalizations. My entire thirties were a decade I would like to forget, ten crummy years with more bad than good.

I wanted a meaningful and lasting relationship. By then, I didn't even know how to meet someone, so I answered personal ads in the local papers. Amazingly, I never had a negative or creepy experience with these dates, but nothing lasted. Then one afternoon, in a local restaurant bar, I met a guy who seemed like a lot of fun. There was a definite spark, and after a few months of seeing each other, he moved into my house. I soon realized I was living with an alcoholic. Even stranger, the moment he moved in he literally never touched or spoke to me. He became a recluse, just sitting in the basement drinking — it was weird.

It was hard to break up with him because his family was so supportive. They took me on their boat every weekend and were fun, good people. They kept me in their home when I had surgery, while my own family never even visited me in the hospital — even when they knew I was hurting.

Soon after he moved out, I lost my 20-year job with Liberty Mutual. I was hospitalized once again. The depression was bad enough for another round of electroshock treatments.

When I was released, I searched for a job but soon found my skills were not very marketable. My knowledge and experience were too specific. Fortunately, I received a good severance package and was able to pay off my mortgage. Expenses were low, but I needed a job to structure my days. A few months later, my old boss called and offered me my old job back. I immediately accepted.

Things were stable for the next few years, but the work was dull. Four of us were doing work three people could easily handle. The job lasted three years until my entire department was let go. We were told our jobs were eliminated due to new computer software. Later, I discovered the company never implemented the new technology — I felt angry and betrayed.

During the final years with Liberty, I met a Paul, a wonderful man who became my husband. He lived in my neighborhood; his former wife actually introduced us. But even though everything else was stable and good, I had another bout with depression. Paul and I spent hours talking. *"Why is this happening to me?"* I thought if I, or we, could find the reason, then I could find the solution. But there was no reason, no magical insight that would bring a cure. I had a chemical imbalance in my brain. My mother had the same problem; so did her mother, who committed suicide before I was born. Neither was my father's side immune to mental illness. One of my cousins had a breakdown in her early twenties, and another cousin was diagnosed as bipolar and died when he was forty from the disease and the alcoholism that shadowed the mental illness.

There was no reason, no rationale; there was only a disease.

During this same time, Mom relapsed into a depression and never recovered. She died of heart failure. I am sad that her life was so difficult. She was locked in so many fears. Yet, despite her illness, she was a good and kind person. When she was well, she had a sharp sense of humor, a quick mind, and was always easy to talk to — I miss her terribly.

Two years later, my father died, another kind of heart failure — he simply lost his will to live after my mother died. Dad was proud of me, proud that I did well in school and had lots of friends. He believed I was strong, and he never thought "it" would happen to me. When I got sick, I felt I'd let him down. It must have been painful for him to see me suffer in the same way as Mother. I wish he could have lived to see how well my life turned out.

As I entered my forties, I was in a stable, loving relationship, but I needed a career to fill out my life. It was not easy this time. I filled out applications, sent resumes, called everyone I knew who might possibly have a lead. I got up every morning, but I felt there was nothing to do. When I was working, I had also enjoyed volunteering. So, I began to serve food at a shelter for the elderly and work with children at a school for students with problems. I did not tutor the students; we were mainly buddies, eating lunch with the kids and just being their friends. But it was not enough. I am a person who needs, who literally depends, on a career to channel my energy.

As the job search became more difficult, I began to have physical symptoms with the growing depression and anxiety. When I filled out an application, my hands shook so terribly that my writing was illegible. Once, I was at a copy shop trying to fill out a cover sheet for a resume I was faxing.My hands were shaking so uncontrollably that I dropped the form. A man who worked at the shop saw what was happening and filled the form out for me — I was grateful.

Finally, I talked to a neighbor, who advised me to change physicians. Since I wasn't getting any better, it seemed like good advice. From the beginning, I felt good about my decision to see Dr. Sethi. He spent more time with me during our first session than any previous doctor had. The only test I couldn't understand was when he asked me to count backward by sevens and threes. I thought, "A lot of people couldn't do this no matter what their mental health." However, with follow-up visits, I felt more confident as I was doing better with the serial sevens and threes.

He tried several medications. One made me feel much better, but it severely affected my depth perception. The first week, I backed into a mailbox and bumped a tree. Dr. Sethi was reluctant to change my medications again because I was feeling so much better, but he said he did not want me bumping into anything else. After trying several, we found a combination that worked — really worked. The fear, anxiety, lack of focus, trembling, and depression began to melt away.

I found a new job in less than a month after the prescriptions began to take affect. A year later, I felt bold enough to apply for a position that is far more challenging and offers an opportunity for growth.

I feel respected in my career for the first time in years. I am relaxed and comfortable in most situations. Paul and I were married when I was forty-three by a Humanist minister. We never seriously considered having children. He felt too old to be a decent father for a young child, and I had serious doubts about passing my genetic soup to another generation.

I have never felt better. I do not know what the future holds, but neither do I fear it. I lay down at night fearing neither consciousness nor death. I do not think of the bad times very much, just occasional shadows, wondering if "*it*" will ever return. But in this moment, I am free to settle where I will. Most of all, *I am grateful* for the life I am living—now, today.

PSYCHIATRIC ASSESSMENT

I have often told my patients that if the "god of psychiatry" came into my office—gave an apparently sound diagnosis and then asked me to write a prescription for a patient—I would be reluctant to comply. It is not that I do not revere the mysterious or distrust the scientific method; it is that no diagnosis and treatment is sound if it does not resonate with your own experience and knowledge of each patient's uniqueness. You have to know the patients' stories, their previous diagnosis, treatments, and they must trust your knowledge and care. It is with this caution that I began to form Betsy's diagnosis and treatment.

Betsy came into my office in July of 1999. Her hands were shaking so severely that she had been unable to drive herself.

She was living with her boyfriend, Paul. He was concerned about her condition and appeared supportive and caring. Betsy's presenting symptoms were hand tremors, general nervousness, and drowsiness. Betsy felt physically weak, depressed, fearful, and tired. When feeling well, she said, she enjoyed hard work, but she had been laid off her 20-year position with her company in the spring. Since then, her condition had deteriorated, she was lethargic and had little motivation. Paul helped with the groceries, partially because Betsy was unable to make simple decisions such as what to wear and what to cook at home. However, Betsy did feel comfortable going to stores and restaurants. One of the critical issues was Betsy's inability to focus and concentrate. She was alert, oriented to the day of the week, the month and year, but she was not sure of the date. To access the severity of her disorientation, I asked Betsy the name of her city and state, her home address, and telephone number. She was able to remember these with ease. She was asked to name the last four U.S. presidents backward in the right sequence, starting with the present one. She had significant difficulty and made errors. She also made errors in subtracting seven from 100 and continuing with this series. Likewise, she made errors in subtracting three from 20 and continuing with the series. This suggested serious problems with her focus and attention.

While Betsy said she had occasional suicidal thoughts, she had not made any specific plans to hurt herself. Neither did she have any homicidal thoughts. She denied any obsessions or compulsions, such as repetitive hand washing, being afraid of germs, checking door locks several times, putting things in perfect order, or performing any rituals. She did not suffer from hallucinations, paranoia, delusions or emotional outbursts, nor did she abuse alcohol, smoke marijuana or cigarettes, or use illegal drugs. As Betsy began to talk, her speech was quite slow and nervous. However, she was friendly, pleasant, and made good eye contact. Betsy is five feet, six inches tall, physically fit, and weighed 155 pounds. She was well dressed in a long black skirt with a matching blouse. Nevertheless, she appeared poorly groomed, with little attention to the details of her physical appearance. Most striking was her pale and very sad face; she carried a look of hopelessness and resignation.

Betsy had good insight into her mental illness. She gave me a detailed history of her several hospitalizations, electroshock therapies, and the medications she had been treated with. When she was 30, and not taking any medications or abusing drugs, Betsy had a single manic episode when she experienced grandiose feelings, believing she was the manager of her department, possessed the energy to do anything, and needed little sleep. At the time, she was also over-spending, buying useless items she neither wanted nor needed. She also believed she was receiving special messages from the television and radio meant just for her. After this episode, she was hospitalized and diagnosed with Bipolar Affective Disorder.

She shared her family's history of mental illness, which was present on both her mother's and father's side. Betsy also told the story of her childhood, family life, and relationships.

She was not suffering from any other medical illnesses, nor taking any other medications or over-the-counter drugs. She was taking Zyprexa 5 mg at night, two Depakote 500 mg in the morning and evening, and Alprazolam 0.5 mg per day on as needed for anxiety. She had been prescribed Lithium but had side effects. She had also taken antidepressant medications but could not recall their names.

Based on her presenting symptoms, I concluded her shaking, poor focus, memory problems, and lethargy were side effects of possible overmedication from taking Depakote (a mood stabilizer) 1000 mg twice a day. Unsure if I would be able to secure Betsy's former psychiatric records, I presented her a working diagnosis of Bipolar Affective Disorder with depressed mood, Generalized Anxiety Disorder, and side effects from Depakote. I recorded her strengths as hardworking, successful, a visibly kind person who had a supportive and loving friend.

This, or any, diagnosis does not exist is some perfect rational vacuum. Like every physician's judgment, it is affected by his training and research in the field of specialization. This is especially true in psychiatry.Depending on when and where psychiatrists were trained and worked in their residency programs, there can be wide variations in diagnosis and treatment. Prior to the mid 1980s, and the gradual acceptance of *DSM III* and DSM *IV's* diagnostic criteria, there were two broad schools of psychiatry—biological and psychoanalytical. Depending on the medical school and particular views of the mentoring psychiatrist, students and new physicians were heavily influenced to side with one of these schools.

I requested, but did not receive Betsy's former medical records. However, one has to be careful in interpreting the diagnosis of other professionals. Psychiatrists trained in psychoanalysis generally do not tell their patients their diagnosis, fearing it may affect a patient's perception and reaction to treatment. Psychoanalytic psychiatrists also may not prescribe medications. As the biological diagnostic criteria of *DSM III* and DSM *IV* are now almost exclusively recognized, this radical difference in treatments is slowly disappearing.

I then educated Betsy and Paul about her diagnosis and the medications. She was taking Depakote (a mood stabilizer) 1000 mg twice a day along with Zyprexa, (a second generation antipsychotic medication, which is also useful for mood stabilization) 5 mg at night. In addition, she was taking the anti-anxiety drug Alprazolam (Xanax). It was possible that these medications were given to Betsy while she was hospitalized. The relatively high dosages may have been prescribed to bring her severe psychiatric symptoms under control. It is additionally possible that her Depakote blood level was adjusted to be in the therapeutic range. However, on her first visit to my office, Betsy was exhibiting negative cognitive and behavioral symptoms, which were possible side effects of her medications. The first step I took was to carefully reduce her medications slowly enough that she did not slip into manic symptoms.

I reduced her Depakote to 500 mg in the morning and 1000 mg at night and Alprazolam to 0.25 mg per day as needed for anxiety. The Zyprexa was continued at the same dosage. Betsy and Paul were informed to call me or go to the Emergency Room if she was overwhelmed by suicidal thoughts. They denied having any guns at home. They were advised to discard any medications, such as Lithium, that she was not taking at this time. Together, they were cautioned that Betsy should avoid driving, and because of the reductions in dosages, a follow-up appointment was made within a week.

FOLLOW-UP SESSIONS

Betsy returned seven days after her initial visit. She stated that she was taking her medications as prescribed. She said she was feeling less anxiety and nervousness; however, she was sleeping a lot — about 13 hours each night. There was an occasional smile on her face. She was slightly more alert and less forgetful, though her hand tremors were severe.

Betsy was cautioned about driving. Her Depakote dose was reduced from 1500 mg to 1250 mg, and her Zyprexa dose was reduced from 5 mg to 2.5 mg. Zyprexa is an antipsychotic medication. It is also useful in the management of manic symptoms. Its major side effect is weight gain. Since Betsy did not have had any psychotic symptoms, I decided to reduce its dose. An appointment was scheduled in one week.

During the third session, Betsy reported she was sleeping better and that her memory was starting to improve. Her ability to subtract serial sevens from 100 was slightly improved. Her overall thinking was also becoming clearer. Betsy said, however, that her anxiety continued, and remarked that she had suffered from this nonspecific nervousness throughout her life. She was disappointed that the Social Security disability application she had submitted had been denied and worried her severance income and benefits would run out in two months.

She said her mood was slightly better and denied having suicidal thoughts. I recommended she continue taking the Depakote and Zyprexa at the same doses. Her Alprazolam (Xanax), which was to be taken on an as needed basis was discontinued and substituted with Klonopin, a longer acting antianxiety medication. Her next appointment was scheduled in ten days.

At this session, Betsy drove herself and said that she had started to clean, cook, and do the grocery shopping. Her mood and memory continued to improve. Importantly, her anxiety was lessening, and she reported no manic symptoms. Betsy noted that she was still sleeping excessively. Her Depakote was reduced to 1000 mg per day, and she was taken off Zyprexa. She continued on Klonopin 0.25 mg two to three times per day.

Two weeks later, during her fifth appointment, Betsy said she had become very panicky and nervous during a job interview, so much so that she had not been able to complete the application forms. She was clearly disappointed, tearful, and depressed. She was very worried about her financial situation. Betsy did not recall the names and dosages of the previous antidepressants she had been prescribed, and I had not yet received the medical records from the hospital or from her previous psychiatrists. Betsy did remember a trial prescription of monoamine oxidase inhibitors and mentioned she had been treated with electroshock therapy.

I wanted to be gentle in my approach. While Betsy may have tried Prozac in the past, there was no record and she did not remember taking the medication. I started her on Prozac 10 mg per day for a week, and then raised the dosage to 20 mg along with her Depakote and Klonopin. I also recommended psychotherapy. She was reluctant because of her previous experiences, but she said she would make an appointment with a therapist.

In two weeks, during her next session, she said she had become engaged, and now her worries concerned the wedding, clothes, dresses, guests, the reception, and the expenses. Her memory and mood were improving, and she was able to do serial sevens smoothly without making any mistakes. Nevertheless, she continued to remain quite anxious and worried. Her Klonopin was increased to 0.25 mg three to four times a day. The other medications were continued at the same dosage, and an appointment was scheduled in three weeks.

However, in one week, Betsy called and said the Prozac was not working. She said she was depressed, unmotivated, not eating well, waking up several times during the night, and was suffering from severe hand shaking, which she found very embarrassing. She was given an emergency appointment. At this time, the Prozac was discontinued, and she was started on a low dose of Serzone at night, to be increased every four days until she was taking 200 mg. Serzone is normally recommended by its makers to be taken twice a day. In my clinical experience, most of my patients feel uncomfortably drowsy taking the medication in the morning. Therefore, I advise them to take Serzone only at night.

Her next appointment was in two weeks. At this time, Betsy reported she had driven to New York City to visit her father, who was sick and in the hospital. Her mood and memory were improved, but she continued to be confused at times and was not able to concentrate. Her nervousness and hand trembling continued. She was getting along well with her fiancé and did not have any sexual dysfunction as when she was taking Prozac. Her dose of Depakote was gradually reduced from 1000 mg to 750 mg for two weeks, and then to 500 mg.

Taking 200 mg of Serzone at night, Betsy continued to be drowsy during the day and was having difficulty focusing while she was driving. She had gone for another job interview, and felt very nervous and shaky. She also experienced dizziness when bending down. In view of these symptoms, her dose of Serzone was reduced to 100 mg, and she was started on Wellbutrin SR 100 mg per day. Wellbutrin is chemically related to the stimulant amphetamine. Thus it is a stimulating antidepressant, gives more energy, and it does not have any sexual side effects. While it is not addictive, it should not be taken after 6 PM as it can interfere with sleep. In Betsy's case, I had to be additionally careful with the dosage of the medications so as not to induce any manic symptoms. She continued on Depakote 500 mg at night, along with Klonopin 0.25 mg three times per day.

The following session, Betsy said her father had passed away at 75 of cardiac arrest. She returned to New York with Paul, made all the funeral arrangements, and had no problems. Her handwriting and shakiness were improving, and her driving was better. Under the circumstances, she was doing quite well. As she improved, Betsy decided to discontinue psychotherapy. Meanwhile, I had read a clinical report in the September 1999 issue of *Neurology* that Remeron helped in treating hand tremors. Remeron is an antidepressant that helps patients sleep better and improves appetite. Many patients can gain weight while taking Remeron, so it needs to be closely monitored. Based on this study, I discontinued Serzone and started Betsy on Remeron 15 mg at night, along with Depakote, Wellbutrin, and Klonopin.

After three weeks, Betsy reported that she had gone for a second interview for a job with an insurance company and she was "feeling 100% better." She had no mood swings, her tremors were improving, and her concentration and focus were better. She had lost 5 lbs, and she was starting to do some exercise. Her sleep and appetite were well regulated, and she was looking forward to her marriage.

Her next visit was scheduled in one month. Betsy came to the office stylishly groomed in professional clothes. She was very happy that she was adjusting to her job. People at the office liked her. She was getting along well with her fiancé and had no sexual problems. She was looking forward to Christmas, New Year's Eve, and her upcoming wedding. She was free of any side effects from the medications.

I continued to see Betsy once a month for several months until she and Paul were married. Thereafter, her appointment schedule was once every two months. She earned a promotion at work, and she is building a house with her husband. She is currently taking Depakote 500 mg at night along with Remeron 15 mg, Wellbutrin SR 100 mg in the morning, and Klonopin 0.25 mg three times a day. Betsy says she does not suffer from any side effects from the medications. She lost more weight, reducing to a healthy 145 pounds. Her marriage and work are doing well, and she is very happy with her life.

Betsy is currently on four psychiatric medications at relatively low dosages. This combination has stabilized her symptoms for more than three years. During this time, she has not been hospitalized and is functioning well in her life. Given her chronic illness and the possibility of changes in her employment, health, and other stressors, she will need continual monitoring.

Betsy was helped in having medical insurance that did not interfere with her treatment plan. Unfortunately, there are insurance companies that allow only three to five psychiatric sessions for an entire year, without additional extensive paperwork.

In recent years, there has been a growing rift between managed care companies and physicians. No doubt, much of physicians' annoyance toward the HMOs is because they are being paid less for an ever-increasing workload. No one wants to work more for less income. Yet, the rub is when physicians increasingly feel they are no longer being trusted to provide what they believe is the best care for their patients. This is perhaps more true in psychiatry than in any branch of medicine. When I began my private practice 13 years ago, there were five psychiatric hospitals serving a metropolitan region of two million people. Between 1997 and 1999, three of these facilities closed due to insurance companies denying payments to patients, most of whom truly needed inpatient care. A fourth facility is soon to close for the same reasons.Sadly, this health care issue will increasingly impair the recovery of individual's suffering as well as their families.

As patients switch employment positions (even within the same community), or their employers change insurance companies almost every year, they are forced to change to other physicians because not every doctor is affiliated with every HMO plan. This is a significant factor in eroding further the patient-physician relationship. Sadly, medicine is becoming increasingly "industrialized" as patients become "clients," "customers," or "subscribers" and doctors "providers".

As patients are assigned to physicians by the managed care companies primarily for financial reasons, the ancient and sacred trust between healer and patient is eroding. This is especially detrimental in the mental health care. Thus there is a increasing confusion and frustrations for clinicians and patients as they are shuffled between therapists, social workers, psychologists and psychiatrists.

CHAPTER 3.

Time's Glory

Time's glory is to calm contending kings,
To unmask falsehood, and bring truth to light.
Shakespeare

Cathleen Rutter was my first glory, my first heroine, and my first Cathy. A stiff upper lip, British Canadian — she was our fortress. Slim and slender, she was virtually my twin. As my father's envoy, I sat with my mother Cathleen — never touching — in the back of our friend's car. Bill Partridge, a man who had a heart of gold and a butt of iron, drove alone in the front. There was no hint of indiscretion, as he trooped all the older ladies in town to their doctors and appointments. If Bill had the time, Mother would have taken this 12-mile trip every day. As best as I can remember, we drove about once a month between 1948 and 1949 to the Norfolk State Prison. The man we went to visit was my brother Richard. Fifteen years older, when he wrote to me from the war, he wrote to a child. He went ashore at Normandy on D-Day plus 30, attached to heavy artillery 155 Howitzer battery.

Mainly, he drove a truck on the Red Ball Express, which was the main supply line for the Third Army. As Richard went up and down the Foley Gap to keep Patton's ego well-supplied, he found a bottle of wine at every stop. One photograph stands out. It is from Bavaria; he is sitting in an embroidered chair, dragged out for the occasion, buddies on every side. With bottles raised, they drank their way through Europe. This was the end for my brother. He died fifty years later, either cirrhosis or lung cancer; I'm not sure because those years were my blankness.

All I can touch is a wooden canoe he made for me in prison. We would park, walk to the front gate, and go down a long walkway into the first building. There was a store to the left with goods made by the inmates. Door A would open electronically, then we walked to door B, which opened into the inner, inner sanctum. The visiting building was an open room lined with benches against the walls. There were no plastic walls between families then. Neither were there tears nor hugging from my loving mother, just pure, tough love that always kept things together one more day. Over the years, I lost the canoe he gave me; it is one of my few regrets.

We were born and raised in Arlington. It was called Arlington Heights, because it rises up the hill from Boston. Our home was an 1885 Victorian, with her lace removed, a clabbered slate roof, and a captain's watch fenced in by a railing. Like my father, the harbor had receded away, but you could still see Boston from the watch.

My father was my polar opposite in every way. He hated Catholics, Jews, blacks, and just about everyone else. I have no idea why. Before my memory, he once owned *J. F. Briggs Printing*. Like everything else in his life, it failed because he did not keep up with what he knew best. He was a typesetter in the old style, where fast hands lined each thin metal strip with mirrored letters. My father is one of those letters to me, something entirely familiar from another world, but distant and useless unless I read it backwards trying to understand.

My parents baptized me in my father's Congregationalist Church. It might have been the last time they ever attended. Mother was low church Episcopalian, but for Easter and Christmas we went to one of the high, fancier Anglican churches in the city, the ones with the brass chandeliers, red robes, and 500-pound crosses.

On ordinary Sundays, I went by myself to St. Johns. It was a perfect fit for a ten-year-old boy who felt a need to go because it was the "right thing." Each Sunday, I put on my brother's old suit, rode the "woody" streetcar down the hill into Cambridge, and then took the subway into Boston. Such diligent, meticulous boys were chosen to become acolytes; they did everything decently and in order and never asked why. I loved lighting each candle in its proper place and time, closing the gates, giving out bread, and feeding their faces. Throughout my life, others have seen me as an extrovert, outgoing, and the last to leave the party. There is no greater rush for this old man than riding my bike, a beautiful BMW, until the needle passes 110 on its way to 130. But inside, I have always been that young boy — traveling by himself to a place where everything will be just the same.

My second heroine was Colette, who waited for my brother while he was in prison so they could be married. She was a Martin, everything my father hated — foreign, Catholic. Her father was a giant of a man, a true Boston Irish cop, tough on the job and drunk the rest of the time.

Colette was as real as her mashed potatoes soaked with butter. When she hugged you, you knew it. You felt her care in your bones.

For most of their lives, Colette and my brother Richard lived in a small house in Watsonville, California. Unlike our father, my brother was a hard worker, a construction man and welder, but like Dad, he was never an earner. Colette waited while he spent his entire paycheck before he got home. One night, he came in with several "buddies" at two or three in the morning. Colette hid in the closet holding my nieces, Ann and Cathy, while they beat my brother and took what little money was left.

Richard sobered up the last fifteen years of his life. My last memory of him was fuzzy; I was still drinking. I drove through California and spent some time with a buddy in Palm Springs before I saw Richard in hospice a month before he died. Since we had been together a few weeks before, I decided not to attend his funeral. However, I did carry Colette's casket, while having a full-blown panic attack. Each step along the 100-yard journey from the hearse to the grave, I kept pounding the words through my head, "One more step, you can make it one more step."

Colette loved my brother — an irresponsible drunk — and somehow lived with him without losing herself. She was so real that any mess my brother brought home either did not stick or, if it did, she wove it into the fabric of life to warm the soul. I have managed medical groups and seen enough psychiatrists to know the terminology. The last label I would ever place on Colette is "co-dependent." She was simply real. I am not sure if there is a term that captures her essence; it was a quality of such depth that any word attempting to enclose it sounds almost profane.

My first tour in Vietnam was from November of 1966 until November of the next year. I was separated by distance and love from my new wife, Brigitte. We met when I was stationed in France for three and a half years. Her father was a French aristocrat, with drivers and maids. He was the Commissioner of Insurance, a government title at a sub-cabinet level position. There were weeks of receptions and an enormous wedding. The irony of it is that our marriage was more of a business deal than anything else.

Brigitte is French Catholic and became pregnant with our son Chris while we were dating. Three priests refused to marry us. I didn't even believe in God at the time. As they tried to convert me to Catholicism, it was like arguing with an ancient mariner to sail around the earth when he still believed it was flat. I did not believe in the destination and saw the journey only as painful and dangerous.

Soon after we were married, we were stationed in California. Brigitte returned to France to have our son. A month later, I was on a troop ship.

I ended up in the middle of a jungle. The closest city of any size was Qui Nahon on the coast. The station was inland, 15 miles from a small village named Pha Thanagh. I was assigned the commander of a heavy supply company of 300 men. The unit had four commanders in the previous six months, all who failed. I made it work. It was a time of achievement. My greatest talent is bringing order out of chaos, and yes, it is true we rarely can give ourselves what we grant to the rest of the world.

We worked in the jungle for 15 to 17 hours each day; every night ended with tons of beer until we passed out and started over again. It was so hot that you never urinated; you literally sweated out all your liquids. All except the ones who went through with the malaria pills. Every man was issued malaria pills, and every single one of us got the runs. There was a continuous line to the latrines — four holes in the ground.

My unit was a stunning success; I brought perfect order to the jungle. However, the more I achieved, the more paranoid I became. If I did not hear praise from a commander for a few days, I was sure something was wrong and I would be found out. I thought the paranoia, and then the phobias with their accompanying anxiety attacks, were from the stress of the war. That is, until I came home.

I met our son Chris the day before Thanksgiving. His father was a train wreck. The paranoia was growing worse as I believed that every terrible thing that *could* happen *would* happen. Life grew more terrifying as thoughts lodged in my head: "Is this thing going to occur?" "Is my wife going to die?" But the most terrifying fear for this solider? It was literally that I would crap in my pants. The added irony of it, of course, is that the bowels are one of the first organs to feel anxiety.

Here was a man who earned two Legions of Merit, three Bronze Stars and an Army Commendation Medal, and I was paralyzed by the fear of not being able to find a bathroom. The panic attacks flooded over me whenever I was in a place were I couldn't get out — a bus, theatre, elevator, or leading a thousand men across a parade field, anywhere you could not escape to a bathroom. I self-medicated with at least a bottle of wine or a case of beer, which naturally made me further depressed and entrapped.

During this time, I often thought of my brother Richard; realizing he probably felt the same pain in WWII — the stress of keeping up.

Five months after I returned from Vietnam, Brigitte's sister was visiting from France. With the added stress of extra family, we both knew it would never work. I was sitting on the toilet (appropriately) when I looked at Brigitte and said, "I think we need to take a break." With Chris, the four of us drove to the airport. We never lived together again. We were separated for almost five years until I received an embossed, wax-sealed letter written in French telling me that we were officially divorced. We remain as we began — friends. Brigitte and I stay connected through occasional phone calls and letters. Chris lives in France; we enjoy each other and talk often, but he likes his silence more and remains unmarried, unattached, and a bit of a recluse.

The Army sent me to the University of Georgia in Athens, where I received a master's degree in Business Administration. The drinking just got worse, but now I was taking Librium and Valium for the paranoid-driven anxiety. I was miserable, shaking, and pathetic.

My second tour in Vietnam was in 1971. For Americans, it was the beginning of the end of the war. Again, I was able to bring order out of chaos. My job was to design and command a unit to take down all the major communication facilities in the country. The identical, long days, the worries if I was doing everything right, worsened the drinking and stress with all the old symptoms. Being in war did not alter my old patterns, it just hardened them.

From 1968 until 1972, I took the deceptive and easy path. I started seeing social workers and taking occasional casual doses of "Benzos." Of course, that did not interfere with my drinking — God forbid.

The one thing that has remained constant in my life is the value I give to the truth. Our honest self is the greatest gift we can give to another. If there has been any glory I chased through time, it was to unmask deceit and to chase truth out in the open. Honesty is the first mark of an officer and a gentleman. Far more important, the love of truth is what makes us human.Looking back on these years, I feel more humor than contempt or pity for the solider who was honest about everything except his drinking.

Drinking was a blast sometimes, but sobriety brought a new kind of misery each morning. Every day I was telling myself, *"Stop!"*

Returning home as a lieutenant colonel, I was accepted into an elite unit at Ft. Lee and attended the Commander General College. It was the first time I saw a psychiatrist. Knowing that going to a military physician would be placed on my record, I saw a private doctor in town. He diagnosed me as manic-depressive, and prescribed Mellaril and Elavil. The drugs took the edge of the symptoms, and for the first time, I started to recover. But the drinking never stopped; it was "my medicine." Later in the year, a new psychiatrist prescribed Triavil for anxiety and depression. I felt better, if you don't count the hangovers. I prayed to a God that I hardly believe in, begging Him to help me make it through the day and survive the pounding in my head. Thankfully, He never stopped the hangovers.

I met my third heroine, Kathleen, while "medicating" at an officers' club. For years, we joked that we got married so I would have a driver to take me home from parties. I did need her protection, but Kathy was the first person I ever loved. She taught me the value of touch. It is a thing the soul needs to survive — to touch and be held.

Kathy introduced me to my fourth heroine, her mother, Florence. Her husband was a senior executive with one of the nation's largest banks and flat-out one of the meanest men I've ever met. Not long after Florence died, Kathy and I were visiting from North Carolina. With just a glance, her father turned to me and said, "I find you boring, dull, and uninteresting." Well, I found him a little repetitive. Even though I didn't like myself most of the time, I wasn't about to have a banker tell me I was tedious. I went upstairs and packed my suitcase as Kathy asked me what was going on. I told her, and she took my hand as we walked out together. The sadness was that such a thing never would have happened if Florence had been alive. She simply wouldn't have allowed it.

In spite of her husband's domineering cruelty, Florence managed to raise three kind and beautiful children. She made bricks without straw, creating a loving family by herself. By the time I met her, she had given up on life, spending her days by herself, reading. Yet, even then she had enough strength to welcome me as another son. I still talk to her picture; it is a focal point, an icon, a window into a place where kindness is stronger than cruelty.

In 1973, Kathy and I came to a branch in the road. I was told I would be a full colonel soon, and making general was a real possibility. However, those positions meant greeting lines, parties, and speaking in confined places. We knew I couldn't survive with my phobias and anxiety, so together we decided to leave the Army. We envisioned another 20-year career of successes as I took a position with Ingersol-Rand in New Jersey.

I was assigned to be a project manager building and designing distribution centers, but everything fell apart in less than a year. I was still drinking, and with the new stress, the phobias and anxieties returned. I was terrified someone thought I wasn't doing my job well, so I worked and drank even harder. The company had an in-house resource, the "Employee Assistance Program." Their slogan was, "If you need help, come see us." I did, and the next week I found myself sitting in front of a computer, playing Solitaire.

I knew there was no future for me with the company, so I asked for a decent severance and walked away. This is when I began to crash. In my old style of working harder and longer than anyone else, I sent out 3,000 resumes. Only one answered — it was a hand-written letter from the founder and president of Food Lion; he was sorry that he could not hire me at the time.

I began working minimum wage positions — a greeter in a department store, a clerk. One day I was in a freight elevator and fell to my knees crying.

I had been seeing Dr. Sethi for two years. The first line in my chart quotes me saying, "I feel like a boy who has not matured into a man, and feel less than others." I probably felt those words, but their memory is lost in a haze of anxiety, depression, phobias, but more than anything else — the lie. As with every other psychiatrist, when Dr. Sethi asked me if I drank, I said I had a glass of wine with dinner "every now and then." What I didn't tell him was that the wine was before and after I had already drained a half a bottle of Scotch.

St. Augustine said the only thing that shall vanquish is truth, and the victory of truth is kindness. But first there is the pain and anger. Three months before I was forced to tell the truth, I wrote a letter to Dr. Sethi blaming *him* for my trouble.

Please stop trying to maintain me at an "almost-well" level. I am not at that level. To help you, my daily feelings are: waves of fear, nausea, a stiff neck and back, desperation, lack of drive, and extreme fatigue after times of stress.

I admire you and the sincerity with which you have tried to help me. I must say, however, that if you refuse to recognize the level of my difficulties, I will be forced to find someone who will. I don't want to do that. HELP!

There is no healing or kindness without truth. Dr. Sethi couldn't treat symptoms enclosed in a lie. Yet, there was still love. I was sitting in my chaise lounge working on my seventh or eighth Coors Light. The same routine every day: I would start drinking at noon and not stop until I went to bed. This day was different. Kathy and my beautiful 14-year-old daughter, Susan, walked down the stairs and said, "Make a choice, either us or the booze." Kathy made the phone call. Sitting bent over in a heap on Dr. Sethi's sofa, the next morning I told the truth about my drinking for the first time in 32 years.

The ragged edge of truth is that it forces us to make decisions. These were mine: no wife, no daughter, and no more treatment until I went to AA and dried up my old butt. It was March 27, 1994. It is easy to remember your birthday.

At first, I thought AA was a bunch of "bull," but thanks to these people, I began to grow up and see life as it was. True spirituality began to seep into my life. Today, I call myself a Christian and try with absolute faith to live as Christ lived, following in his ways, though falling down most of the time.

The journey back was not easy. Stopping drinking was only the first step. I have never had a drop since that night, and only once was I even tempted. We were eating with friends at a bar that reeked of beer. I said that I needed to leave, and because they were friends, they were happy to go to another place.

The rough part of the road home was changing my behavior. I had to become a new person and see the world from a completely different place. It was not easy, especially finding a decent job. I sorted clothes hangers, was a "bug man" for a couple months, and tried to sell a worthless product for a few months more. Eventually, things grew better. Today I am the senior administrator of the largest mental health practice in the area.

Yes, I am still able to command order in the midst of chaos. Unless it is my own mess; then I need a lot of help. Am I perfect? No, I just don't drink and so I have clearer eyes and a stronger mind to face the fears and anxieties knowing I cannot make it alone.

Thanks to all of you who have loved me along the way.

Psychiatric Assessment and Follow Up

Alcohol and drug abuse have been prevalent in almost every society. Among those who suffer mental illness, more than two thirds abuse drugs and alcohol, often in an attempt to self medicate the pain of their psychiatric symptoms. It is likely he was treating his life long symptoms of anxiety, depression, and mild paranoia with alcohol.

Frank is but one of many who have tried to salve the pain of illness through drug and alcohol abuse. Like many individuals, he has a genetic predisposition to alcoholism. Frank is a 52-year-old, white, married professional. When he came into my office on

February 24, 1992, he was well dressed and appeared physically fit — six feet two inches tall and 182 pounds. Referred by a local psychiatrist treating his wife, Frank's presenting symptoms were dizziness, fatigue, insomnia, and a general feeling of being stressed and anxious. Frank said he occasionally experienced panic attacks and often was overcome by fear.

For the past six to seven months, he had been taking Xanax 0.5 mg (as needed) and Trazodone 100 mg to help him sleep. In 1991, he was prescribed Prozac 20 mg, but he discontinued it due to adverse side effects. Before that, he had been treated for ten years with Triavil, which is a mixture of the antipsychotic medication P*erphenazine* and the antidepressant A*mitriptyline*. Frank also had been treated with Mellaril and Elavil for some time.

He had relocated from New Jersey to Charlotte as Logistic Distribution Manager with a Fortune 500 company, managing a budget of $20 million. Frank served in the Army for 20 years, earning an MBA while in service and retired as a lieutenant colonel. He and his wife, Kathy, are happily married and have a teenage daughter. Kathy is a college graduate and is supportive of her husband. Their marriage is one of his greatest strengths.

Obviously, in stressful condition such as his tours of duty in Vietnam, Frank decompensated and had to be hospitalized. Decomposition is literally the process of an element separating or breaking-down of something into its basic elements, its decays and disintegrates. The popular term of having a "break down" to describe a person's mental collapse is actually a rather accurate description of what occurs when a victim decompensates—their mind literally beaks down.

During our initial session, Frank described himself as "a child who has not matured into a man," and said he "felt less than others." He was paranoid that people were talking about him and that he was not meeting their expectations. These symptoms were periodic and chronic. While stationed in Vietnam, Frank was hospitalized in a psychiatric ward, diagnosed as having Manic Depressive Disorder.As Frank never had a single manic episode, his initial diagnosis of Manic Depressive Disorder by military psychiatrists in the 1970's may have been misleading. In an attempt to be more specific in the 1980's, DSM III and DSM III R in the 1980's began using the term "Bipolar Disorder" to describe patients who have at least one manic episode or alternate between episodes of depression and mania.

Following a thorough physical examination by an internist (including a full blood workup), Frank was diagnosed as having a spastic colon, which causes intermittent abdominal pain and loose stools. There were no abnormalities in the blood work.

Frank stated he used to drink heavily in college and in the military, and that he was currently drinking one to two beers a night, "and a few more on weekends while watching ball games." Based upon my observations and his presenting symptoms, my diagnosis was that Frank suffered from a Major Depressive Disorder, Generalized Anxiety Disorder, Paranoid Delusional Disorder, and possible alcohol abuse.

In view of these findings, I started treating Frank on an anti-anxiety medication, an antidepressant, and a low dose of Haloperidol (0.5 mg) at night. His symptoms did not improve. He continued to undermine his progress by denying his excessive drinking. His work stress increased when he was given a position that Frank said "bored him to death." Additionally, he had no libido. Given these symptoms, he was treated with Wellbutrin, Yohimbine, and Cyproheptadine without success. Prior to Viagra, Yohimbine and Cyproheptadine were used for male sexual dysfunctioning with limited success.

Frank's symptoms of depression escalated. He admitted strong suicidal feelings and had easy access to firearms. In view of this immediate danger, Frank entered a psychiatric hospital in October 1992 for two weeks. During this time, it became clear that Frank was alcohol dependent and had been treating his life-long anxiety and mild paranoia with alcohol.

Ethanol or alcohol is a cytotoxic agent, meaning that, depending on its concentration, it can kill all biological cells. For years, clinicians and researchers used alcohol to sterilize a wound or experiment field. It does the same thing in the blood, essentially killing cells, usually initially destroying liver and brain cells, which are among the first cells to show damage from alcohol abuse.

After being released from the hospital, Frank continued outpatient therapy with a substance abuse counselor. During this time, he did not respond to Wellbutrin or Zoloft, but continued on Navane, Trazodone, and (as needed) Lorazepam. Yet, he refused to reduce his drinking and resisted attending Alcohol Anonymous meetings. With an increasing threat of being fired from work, Frank escalated his drinking and became further depressed. Finally, he lost his job in August 1993.

As alcoholics often drink to self-medicate their anxiety, diagnosis is further complicated as alcohol withdrawal can mimic anxiety symptoms. Because of the additional stigma and guilt surrounding alcoholics, this makes mental illness masked with substance abuse exceedingly difficult to diagnosis. Patients and their families must be totally honest and truthful in sharing their symptoms and behavior.

Frank's medical insurance and severance pay lasted only until the end of the year. In desperation, he accepted a minimum wage job at a local department store earning $5.50 an hour. He then worked for a slightly higher wage at a hardware store. Unable to find a challenging skilled position, Frank felt humiliated and saw his life as a failure. His depression deepened when a business plan with a friend from church did not materialize. Franks' alcohol abuse escalated until he was drinking a gallon of wine a day. He felt tired, utterly discouraged, and had no courage to live; Frank knew he was in immediate danger of losing his beloved wife, daughter, and home. Until Frank became sober, no mediation could help him.

Frank's physical symptoms of nausea, diarrhea, stiffness of neck and back muscles, and extreme fatigue continued to worsen. At this point, I immediately arranged a family session with his wife. He was given the option of going back to the hospital or to an intensive outpatient program for alcohol and drug treatment, which would include attending AA meetings.

It was a life-saving miracle when Frank stopped drinking on March 27, 1994 and started going to AA meetings four to five times per week. He found excellent support in AA, and received a very good sponsor. He continued to work hard on his sobriety and started going to church.

Based on Frank's history, I concluded that he had suffered from Generalized Anxiety Disorder his entire adult life. His depression may have been related to psychosocial stressors as well as to his drinking. He may also suffer from a mild Paranoid Disorder whose symptoms are also exaggerated with alcohol and stress.

Frank responded well to Zoloft (an antidepressant) 100 mg twice a day along with Diazepam (an anti-anxiety medication) 10 mg three times a day. In March 1995, when his job and family situation improved, he was taken off of Zoloft, and the dosage of Diazepam was reduced. Diazepam is the generic name for benzodiazepine family of medications, known as Valium. A low dose of diazepam proved successful because it reduced his general anxiety, making it possible for him to remain sober during stressful times.

Frank moved to a smaller house. He continued family therapy to deal with anger among his family members, particularly his daughter. He also became more involved in church. After several experiments with different jobs, he finally found a challenging job where he could use his talents. Later, he received a significant promotion. His daughter married.

Frank's dose of Diazepam was reduced to 10 mg twice a day. He has been free of anxiety, paranoia and depressive symptoms. His physical symptoms have disappeared. He is very happy with his family and job. He has a great sense of humor. Frank continues therapy once every three months in my office for the past five years.

CHAPTER 4

Too Deep for Tears

Thanks to the human heart by which we live,
Thanks to its tenderness, its joys, and fears,
To me the meanest flower that blows can give
Thoughts that often lie too deep for tears.
William Wordsworth

Deep, unspeakable suffering
may well be called baptism,
a regeneration,
the initiation into a new state.
George Eliot

Singers and artists ask the most heroic and cruelest of deeds. It is to shed our reality for a moment and enter their worlds. For those who have not learned the deep art of suffering, this may not sound like a difficult journey. We watch *Star Wars*, and, for a few moments after we leave the theater, we are Jedi warriors driving our cars through the night. Then we come home, lie in our beds, and another world softly returns a familiar certainty. But, what about those who have been leaving their reality for years and have no place to re-enter?

I had just moved out of a group home in Austin, Texas. The love of my life was a beautiful, blond freshman at the University of Texas. Chip and I met at the *Gap,* where I worked. I was 18, and he was the lust of my life. He was going to college and had a lot in front of him. I told him I wouldn't force him into something he wasn't ready for. It was both our faults, and I wound up carrying the load.

I began working in massage parlors and then a nude modeling agency. They were just covers for prostitution. It was about five months until it was obvious I was pregnant and had to quit, yet the time seemed endless. I would focus on a corner of the room, spacing out and pretending my physical body was doing this but I wasn't. There was only one time I could not flee through my imagination to another reality. He was a huge, sweaty, pimply guy with a big nose. When he was on top of me, I started to cry. He said, "I love it when you cry; it turns me on when you cry."

Out of money and hope, I moved back to Chicago. When my mother saw me, she wouldn't let me stay at her house. She said I had made my bed, now I can sleep in it. After flopping from place to place, I called an adoption agency. They placed me with a family, where we stayed until Anastasia was born. I named her after my sister Stacy. The family was very religious, no TV, always saying, "The Lord did this." They were strict but good people. I spent three days with Stacy in the hospital, then I saw her a week later when she left with her new mother and father and a new name. Though I knew it was for the best, a piece of my soul left with her.

I was three or four when I saw my first psychiatrist. It might have been the last time I was completely sane (whatever that means); it certainly was the end of my innocence. I remember the inkblot and word association tests, wondering, "Why am I having to do this?" Later, I learned the only reason I was at the psychiatrist was so my mother could prove that my schizophrenic father was damaging me so the judge would cancel his visitation rights.

Mom left Dad and moved in with a neighbor five long blocks away from where we had lived. There were two or three times when I defied my mother and rode my bike to Dad's house. He always cried when he saw me. One of my few memories was that he made wooden birdcages. He called me "Tiffy," and there was nothing I could do that was wrong in his eyes.

He was not a saint. My only full sister, Mary Lynn, is mentally retarded and passed through childhood in a series of body casts for scoliosis. Dad saw her as an abomination and said she "couldn't be his child." But I was, and he was the only person who ever gave me unconditional love. I don't try to understand why he couldn't accept Mary Lynn. As a child, I resented the extra attention she received, felt embarrassed by her presence during adolescence, but I would tear a neighborhood kid apart if anyone teased her. Today, she lives in a group home. We talk about once a month and still get together for vacations with our mother. Mary Lynn is much like her father who refused to claim her — not "normal" by the world's standards, but in her own way a bundle of unconditional love.

At least my father was gentle. My stepfather was a brutal drunk. After drinking, he would chase the children through the house and beat whomever he caught. Mainly he hurt the boys, but we all caught the cruelty of his verbal abuse. Like a co-dependent being drawn to alcoholics, I have been unconsciously drawn to these kinds of men all my life. I do not feel like a victim, far from it, but there is something that blindly leads me to these men.

The last time I was in the hospital was shortly after my "millennium crash." The mania began as I waited for the zeros to turn over. I was sure something important was going to happen; I believed God was going to use me in his inevitable transition of the world. At first, I spent summer days getting something accomplished or relaxing with the animals in my back yard. I would sit on a stump and throw the ball to my deaf Dalmatian while I reflected on life. Things had to change; they were going to get better.

The mania deepened, everything was go, go, go as I worked ever more hours. However, I knew at the new millennium, everyone would be enlightened to a higher level, there would be no poverty, no lawsuits, and love would spread throughout the world. Looking back, I am not sure which thought was the most absurd.

When the new millennium came and nothing happened, the thin wall between fantasy and reality disconnected. I could rarely hear a song or watch a movie without becoming detached. I was watching an Arthurian movie, *The Rock and the Sword*; and as the sword was taken from the rock, I became part of the movie and was pulling out the sword as lightness, light, and magic swirled around me. I was watching the movie *Matrix*, and things shifted again; I was part of the movie, disconnected from the world beyond the reality of the screen. Then I was in the back yard, playing scrabble with my husband John, and all his words echoed with evil, while mine had to do with goodness. I heard footsteps and sensed someone was standing over me. These sensations returned several times a week.

Things grew worse. I started picking and scratching my skin. The problem existed for several years. I was obsessed with getting rid of every bump and imperfection. The problem was that my fingernails were like razors, and I would rip and tear my skin until infections set in. Each wound represented an issue or problem. My skin worsened as society grew sicker. I wanted so much to fight for what is right, to solve the world's problems, to set people straight. Sometimes all the little things in life can suddenly pull together to mean something bigger than you could ever expect. Once again, I found myself on this edge of coalescence where the movements of the cosmos were somehow reflected in the coincidences of my day-to-day life.

But when expected mystical events do not occur, there is no place to return, and so like a ghost caught between the spiritual and physical, you are not sure which reality you belong in. To one looking in from the outside, the mania and delusions took over.

When they came to get me, my personal sensation was of giving birth to myself as I lay in bed. John woke in the night and felt wetness on the other side of the empty sheet. My son Mark and husband found me on the front porch. In my consciousness, I was still in my bed. They tell me it took five EMTs to strap me down. They carried me away spitting and cursing.

I was happy to be back in the hospital. It was a place where I felt safe and had a role. I began to reach out to people. I helped other patients discard their shells so they could attend group therapy and activities. I felt as if I actually helped a few people. The day I left, they clapped for me.

When I was around five, my sister Mary Lynn and I were living with my mother, stepfather, and his four children — two boys and two girls. Ricky was eight or nine when we began touching each other. When I was about ten, we were playing Spin the Bottle in a fort, a big old refrigerator box on the edge of our yard next to a church parsonage. There was only one time when there was penetration; it stopped when my stepfather's eyes peered through holes in the box and he yelled, "Knock it off!"

As a child who felt out of place, I admit I enjoyed the warped interest my stepbrothers gave me, even though I knew there was something deeply wrong. Then one day during lunch hour in the junior high cafeteria, this boy stood up and shouted, "Hey Tiffany, did you f _ _ k your bother today?" I am not sure how he found out. I think my stepsister spread the rumors, because in some bizarre way she was jealous of the attention I received from her brothers and felt bad about her own chubby appearance.

From that day in the cafeteria, I was bad news to myself and a joke to the rest of the students. My friends became the "stoners." To fit in, I started smoking pot and taking speed. With so many problems at home and school, I ran away when I was 13. The first time was just for a few days. I stopped by a friend's house, she called my parents, and a cop pulled me from a bus stop to the police station.

The second time, I was away for two weeks. I stayed next to a doorway at an elementary school to keep warm in the snow of a Chicago winter. One night, I was sleeping in the schoolyard when an old friend found me and just held me all night. The next day, his older brother Bob said I could stay at their house, but there was a small price: I had to have sex with him. I lost my virginity and another piece of myself. The whole thing was gross, painful, and I cried silently, feeling shitty that I had stooped this low. However, it was a low with a strange feeling of power. Even though I felt worthless, I recognized the one powerful asset I did possess. Ever since, I have used sex as leverage to get something I want; though I still yearn to be gently embraced, safely held, and touched.

From the schoolyard, it was a series of group homes after a failed attempt to stay with my older half sister from my mother's first marriage. Debby had children of her own, and we were both too young to take care of each other.

The first group home was a big old house with a huge basement. It was only a holding place until there was room in the lock-in treatment center.

The Center was a cold, gray place. The doors were huge; I remember the metal screens in the windows so you could not escape from your bedroom. There was one little window in the

TV room that opened to the outside. We would gather around it to breathe in the fresh air.

Again, I used my sexuality to be accepted. I knew flirting would get me in trouble, but I needed the attention it brought. I was constantly being put off co-ed (no communication with boys).

We had group sessions each day at The Center. One patient would sit in front of the other clients gathered in a half circle behind the one being "treated." There were two rows of counselors lined in front of the patients. Once, I had the front seat when one of the nurses said in her down-home, crushing voice, "Honey, you remind me of my pet poodle in heat." Despite my need for attention, my rule-breaking, I was not a dog — I was crushed, angry, and most of all, embarrassed.

I was released to a "special education" school for the summer. Even there I was not part of the "in" crowd. They made me feel like a handicapped person who does not have the natural abilities to fit into the normal world. It was so bad that I actually asked to be readmitted to The Center. Anywhere was better than this.

This time, The Center felt like a relief; somehow, I felt safe there. It was far from home, but I knew I didn't want to return to my family. The doctors thought I would do better in a long-term facility and let me choose one of three hospitals. I chose Austin, Texas. Old patterns repeated; soon I was off co-ed and restricted to my assigned house. I slowly earned privileges as I began to become healthier. After a year and a half, I passed my high school equivalency exam (GED) and was released. However, by myself, I was out of control; I went through more men than I had treatment centers.

My first serious love was Chip, the blond University of Texas guy. After Anastasia was born, I received a phone call from a guy in Texas whom I vaguely remembered. Somehow, he had managed to track me down. On the phone, he asked me to marry him. With nowhere to go, I said yes. When I arrived at the airport, I couldn't believe how ugly he was. After a few weeks, I moved in with a neighbor in the same apartment complex.

Perry was my next love. I was having sex with a number of different men, and so when I became pregnant again, I wasn't sure if the baby was Perry's or not. He offered to marry me, but he never said he loved me. I told him I loved him with all my heart, and it was important that I knew he loved me back. He left for a one-month float (sea duty), and I got scared. I grabbed on to a regular guy at the bar and asked him to marry me. He was elated, but it was a terrible, short-lived decision. I left a week after we were married. Of course Perry was very hurt by what I did. He later left on a six-month float; I sent so many letters to him telling him I truly loved him, but he never wrote back.

Once again, I knew I did not have the means or stability to be a good mother. I called the same agency in Chicago and asked about the family who adopted Anastasia. They had just applied for a new baby. I wanted the girls to be together, so, once again, I returned to Chicago and moved into a home for unwed pregnant mothers. I stayed at the home throughout the pregnancy and for a brief time afterward. I was able to meet with the adoptive parents and give them my second little girl.Even though it was incredibly difficult, I tried to focus on the better life I was giving them. Though I have never seen either of them again, I know I have two very beautiful girls.

My next mistake with a man was my worst. I went to Jacksonville to find Perry. By the time I found him in a bar, he was already dating another girl. I sat crying in my car as a couple of guys came out and helped me. A few days later, I bumped into one of them at the same bar. Feeling lonely and without a home, I accepted a date. On the second date, we had sex, and despite using contraceptives, I became pregnant again. This time, I committed myself to this baby. Unfortunately, I also made a commitment to his father, a man I hardly new. A Justice of the Peace married us. We were poor. We went fishing as often as possible so we would have decent food. Most of the time, we ate Raman Noodles, chicken broth with rice, and sandwiches.

After we moved to New Jersey, an even tougher reality set in. The man I married was an alcoholic along with being mentally and physically abusive. I felt unable to leave and hoped he would change when Mark was born. The abuse never went away.

We moved to North Carolina, because Richard couldn't find or hold a job and New Jersey had become too expensive to live. I somehow endured his verbal and physical abuse — always followed by countless apologies — for about a year. But the pain was as enduring as the broken promises. Hardly a day passed when he did not tell me that if I left he would hunt me down and kill me.

I left on Easter morning. A week later, Richard found us at a friend's home. Stinking drunk, he grabbed Mark and there was a terrible fight. People finally came out into the street to help me. After a brief stay in a North Carolina hospital, I returned to Chicago, with so little money that I had to give a lady in a toll both an IOU.

Over the next few months, I struggled with being a single parent. I worked two jobs, which meant that Mark was spending ever-longer hours in daycare. One person who watched my son was a close friend of the family; we called him "Uncle John." Then one day my three-year-old son said he and Uncle John were "playing doctor." I almost lost it. We talked with Social Services and went though all the interviews, counseling, and red tape. In the end, we got nowhere. The courts said Mark was too young to testify in court. Later, I learned his abuser had been charged with abuse before but had not been prosecuted.

I ended up moving in with a guy just to help with rent. He was an easy target and really fell for me. We were married, and I found a good job with better insurance. It only lasted a couple of years because I didn't really love him; he was just a temporary fix. I found a better candidate for a husband and father. He was interesting, good-looking, and had a solid work record. Once again, I was living with him in a few weeks, and we were married a year later. My husband John is extremely critical and has a short temper, but at least he is loving, and for a while, life was relatively stable.

John found a job in Charlotte, N.C. I eventually started a job as a personal organizer. Even though my personal life is a mess, I have a natural talent for organizing other people's lives. I help them bring order to messy homes, organizing closets and calendars.

My last manic episode was the one following the new millennium. Since then, my medications have leveled me out. I am now an assistant manager at the largest art store in the city. As long as I remain faithful to my medications, I feel confident that I will not have another breakdown.

Is life normal? For me, it is perhaps as stable as it can be. There is still a thin line between heaven and earth, between the world most people see and the supernatural cosmos of mystics, saints, and lunatics. Besides the medications, I keep stable by talking to a friend I call Bob. I am not sure if Bob is a person, and angel, or both, but I know he is real. He is my soul-mate, the one person I could have a perfect emotional, spiritual, and sexual relationship with; we would be one.

So I work, try to be a good mother to a teenage boy with all the normal troubles and a few extra, and wait for the veil to fold back into another world.

Psychiatric Assessment

Referred by a friend, Tiffany arrived at my office with her husband, John. She asked if her husband could join and help her with the initial assessment. Together, they told her remarkable and harrowing story.

Tiffany was five years old when she first visited a psychiatrist because of stress in her family. By the time she was 13, she said, she was "out of control," using drugs after being sexually abused by her stepbrothers. She was hospitalized in a psychiatric facility for five and a half months in response to the trauma. Tiffany was then sent to a long-term treatment facility for 18 months. When she was 15, she ran away from home and attempted suicide by overdosing on Tylenol. She abused cocaine through her adolescence and used crack from the ages of 17 to 21. Her present marijuana abuse has been sustained for 20 years. Over this time, she also smoked cigarettes, varying from one to three packs of cigarettes per day.

While Tiffany appeared physically fit — 5-foot-5 inches tall, and weighing 130 pounds — she was visibly depressed. She was medically healthy, having had her last physical examination eight months earlier, when she was hospitalized. She has no known allergies, does not take any over-the-counter medications, and takes an oral contraceptive as her only other prescription drug.

A year before this first visit, Tiffany started to compulsively pick the skin on her arms and legs. She went to her primary care office and was prescribed Prozac by a nurse practitioner. The dosage was eventually increased to 60 mg per day. After stopping the prescription, Tiffany deteriorated into what she described as a "nervous breakdown." She felt delusional, received messages from God, had other visions, was overexcited, and had rapid speech. She was hospitalized at a local mental health center for two weeks and treated with Depakote, Paxil, and Klonopin. Her follow-up care consisted of seeing her nurse practitioner on a regular basis. An apparent side effect of the medication was a weight gain of 30 pounds.

Tiffany gradually stopped taking her medications. She described her current symptoms of depression as "having black clouds," no motivation, experiencing crying episodes and a feeling of worthlessness, being unable to function in daily life or at a regular job, increased sleeping and not wanting to get out of bed when she was awake, having no appetite, and wishing she were dead. Tiffany said, however, that she had no plans to kill herself. She denied any obsessions, compulsions, paranoia, hallucinations, delusions or any symptoms of mania. Her memory was intact; her speech was slow but goal-oriented. She continued to smoke marijuana, "because it helps," and was currently smoking up to a pack and a half of cigarettes per day.

Her husband, who has known her for more than five years, said Tiffany has had mood swings throughout their time together. Eighty percent of the time, he said, she is in a manic to hypomanic state, while being depressed only 20%. She also has PMS symptoms five days before her menstrual cycle. On a scale of one to ten, ten being the best and one being the worst, Tiffany rated her overall functioning as "around three."

Tiffany suffered a very painful childhood. She was physically and emotionally abused by her father and sexually abused by her stepbrothers through inappropriate touching. From the age of nine until 16, she was sexually molested and had intercourse with her two stepbrothers, who were two to three years older. When her mother discovered this abuse, Tiffany was hospitalized and her brothers were sent to a treatment facility.

She was born and raised in Chicago and completed her GED in 1985. Her mother, married five times, is 65 years old, and lives in South Carolina. Her biological father died at the age of 76. Tiffany's parents separated when she was five. Her father abused alcohol and drugs and may have had a manic depressive illness. Her sister is mentally retarded, and she has numerous half siblings from several stepfathers.

Between the ages of 17 to 25, Tiffany said she was extremely promiscuous (having over 100 sexual partners) and abused drugs. She gave birth to two daughters during this time; the same family adopted her two daughters. Her first marriage of three years began at the age of 21.

Her 11-year-old son Mark is from this marriage. Currently, she is married to John, who is 45 years old and has a college degree and a stable job. Originally from Hungry, he has lived in the United States for more than 23 years. Tiffany worked in a number of odd jobs and is currently self-employed as a personal organizer for homes and businesses.

She describes her current symptoms as depression and is financially stressed as she is starting her own business. Tiffany's husband and mother continue to be supportive. Her strengths include being street smart, attractive, and a survivor.

Based on these findings, my initial diagnosis was that she has Bipolar Affective Disorder, in a depressed phase, was marijuana and nicotine dependent, and has a history of poly-substance dependence.

Tiffany and John were educated on the psychiatric condition, various medications, and their possible side effects. She was started on Depakote and Paxil. They were counseled to reduce her marijuana and cigarette smoking. I also advised them that Tiffany needed to meet regularly with a psychotherapist and substance abuse counselor, and attend Narcotics Anonymous for additional support.[1] I told them to remove any guns from their home, and said that if her suicidal thoughts should become uncontrollable to go to an emergency room or call my office for a crisis appointment. We scheduled a follow-up visit within ten days.

Follow-up Sessions

Before her second appointment, Tiffany called the office and said that she had nausea at 20 mg of Paxil. I recommended she reduce the dosage to 10 mg. At the second appointment, Tiffany was taking two Depakote 250 mg at night and Paxil 10

---

[1] Narcotics Anonymous (NA) is one of the self-help groups based on Alcohol Anonymous' 12-step program. These groups have enabled millions of people throughout the world maintain sobriety and understand their illnesses. While not a substitute for medications and psychotherapy, they are a vital support for patients, their families, and are invaluable in reducing the chances of relapse.

mg during the day. She was still experiencing nausea and mild diarrhea. She also noted a reduced sexual desire. She appeared slightly more energetic, and her crying and tearfulness were less severe. Her mood was quite depressed and she was mildly anxious, but Tiffany said she had not experienced any further suicidal thoughts. She reduced her marijuana smoking by 20% to 30%, but she had not cut down on the amount of cigarettes. Neither had she seen a therapist nor attended any NA meetings. Her Depakote was increased to 750 mg at night. The Paxil was further reduced to 5 mg, and she was started on a low dosage of Wellbutrin.

When she came in for her session two weeks later, Tiffany was taking Wellbutrin 75 mg twice a day along with the Paxil and Depakote. Her nausea and diarrhea had stopped, and her libido had returned to normal. She complained of a compulsion to scratch and pick the skin over her entire body. Her depression, relationship with John, and new business were all improving. She continued to smoke marijuana and cigarettes with John. Her sleep was better, and I was pleased to see her occasionally smile. I discontinued the Paxil, and she was started on Prozac, while the Wellbutrin SR was increased to 200 mg daily.

A month later, at her fourth session, Tiffany's depression and general feelings showed significant improvement. She had new clients for her business and said she was "feeling 100% better." Her sleep was improved and she was smiling more. However, she was still scratching and picking her skin. Her cigarettes and marijuana use had not slowed. She was given Benadryl and Hydroxyzine to see if they helped her itching. Once again, I strongly urged Tiffany to see a mental health counselor.

Tiffany made an emergency appointment two weeks later; she had stopped all her medications. John had taken two weeks off work to be with her and said her moods were fluctuating between depression, crying, and violent outbursts. She had removed her wedding band and was now cutting her body with nail clippers. Tiffany said she was not suicidal or homicidal and did not want to go to the hospital. She was tearful, dysphoric (a state of marked depression), did not speak, and was withdrawn. She was urged to resume the medications.

There are numerous reasons patients stop taking their medications. The most common is that when patients feel better, often they think they are cured and no longer need drug therapy. Unfortunately, this happens despite educating patients, and their families that psychiatric illnesses are chronic, and thus medications are essential to their ongoing stability and well-being. Various side effects, especially weight gain, reduced sexual functioning and physical symptoms, are other major factors in patients discontinuing drug therapies. Most psychiatric medication can cause these side effects. It is important for patients to know that these side effects are often dose dependent and can be minimized by adjustment of medications. Notorious culprits for weight gain include Zyprexa, Remeron, and Depakote; various serotonin reuptake inhibitors (SRI) such as Prozac, Paxil, Zolft, Celexa, Lexapro and Luvox often cause sexual problems. Thus, at each session, I ask my patients to weigh themselves on an office scale so I can monitor weight changes—as well as ask about any sexual dysfunction—so that I can adjust medications and dosages appropriately.

The following day, John called and said Tiffany was continuing to refuse her prescriptions. Her condition was deteriorating. He said she was "shouting, crying, and out of control." She was further depressed after raccoons killed her cat.

I strongly recommended John to take her to the hospital, where she was involuntarily committed.[2] She spent 16 days at the Community Mental Health Center Hospital under the care of another psychiatrist. She was discharged on Depakote 1500 mg and Risperdal 5 mg per day.

Tiffany had a history of manic symptoms before this most recent hospitalization. Further, her husband described her as fluctuating from high (80% of the time) to low moods (20% of the time). It is not clear to what extent Tiffany's behavior was influenced by poly-substance abuse as well as ongoing abuse of marihuana and cigarettes. Neither is there a fine line between Tiffany's use of these substances to self-medicate and her addictive personality. Nevertheless, after her hospitalization, my initial diagnosis of Bipolar Affective Disorder, type I, with marihuana and nicotine dependence was reaffirmed.

---

[2] Laws for involuntary commitment vary from state to state. Generally, if a person is a danger to self or others, anyone who knows the patient well can go before a magistrate and file a petition for involuntary commitment. Once a petition is filed, the patient is taken by the local legal authorities to the nearest hospital and evaluated by a psychiatrist-physician. If the patient fulfils the local criteria, he or she is then involuntarily committed for treatment.

Tiffany made an appointment with me within a week after being discharged from the hospital. John and her son, Mark, came with her. She said she was very tired and complained bitterly that John was being too critical. John replied that they were not getting along and that she was verbally abusive. He was also worried about a possible relationship she was having with Chad, a 32-year-old patient she met in the hospital, who was taking her to NA meetings. She drank alcohol on Memorial Day and continued to smoke marijuana and cigarettes. She also had gained ten pounds. Tiffany countered her husband's appraisal, saying her mood was improving, the scratching and cutting had stopped, and she was working in the yard planting flowers.

I recommended she consolidate the dosages of Risperdal, taking them only at night. The Depakote was continued at the same dosage. She was advised not to have any contact with Chad and was agreeable to make appointments for individual and family therapy with a psychologist.

Tiffany returned by herself within a week. She spoke of receiving messages from the television and radio and said she was "married to the Antichrist." She was not using the name metaphorically, but literally saw John as the Antichrist. She called the police, telling them that John was drinking with the neighbors. She had met once with Chad and brought him clothes. He was also writing her letters.

She said she was sleeping better and her mood was slightly depressed. Mentally, she had declined, showing difficulty in remembering the last four presidents in sequence. I prescribed

Zyperxa 10 mg at night, and her Risperdal was decreased to 2 mg. Significantly, she had started to visit a therapist.

Tiffany was late at the following session. She said she was still receiving messages from God, who was communicating with her through the television and radio. Her sleep and appetite were better, and her mental ability was improving. She was now working cleaning houses with a friend. Tiffany said she was getting along better with her son and husband and had no contact with Chad.

A week later at her next scheduled session, Tiffany was feeling less paranoid, her messages from God were subsiding, and she had stopped smoking marijuana. Her thinking was clearer, and she said she had not contacted Chad. She was driving by herself and said her therapy was going well. Tiffany added she "had no problems with John or her son." Due to her weight gain, she was agreeable to switch from Depakote to Topamax, thus the Depakote was reduced gradually and substituted with Topamax. Topamax like many anti-seizure medications have proven to be good mood stabilizers. Topamax has the advantage that patients start losing weight.

Tiffany then called within a week and said she was becoming less motivated and depressed. I agreed to her request to start back on Prozac. Two weeks later at her next session, she was taking Prozac 20 mg, Zyprexa 20 mg, Topamax 100 mg twice daily, and Depakote 500 mg. She was more energetic, happy, and was getting along with John and not suffering from frequent highs and lows. The psychotic symptoms were gone, and she received a new job. Tiffany was still smoking two joints of marijuana a day as well as cigarettes. Her Depakote was discontinued, the Topamax was increased to 300 mg, and the Zyprexa was decreased to 15 mg.

I received a call from John who said Tiffany was being dishonest with me and probably was not taking the medications as prescribed. In order to avoid hospitalization, I saw them together the next day. At this session, Tiffany said she was not happy in her marriage, had no sex drive, no motivation, and was growing increasingly depressed. However, she was not suffering from hallucinations, paranoia, or delusions. I added a small dose of Wellbutrin to her other medications and emphasized the importance of continuing with psychotherapy. She scheduled an appointment in two weeks.

In the following monthly sessions, the Welbrutrin SR was titrated gradually and the Prozac reduced to 10 mg. This change helped reduce the sexual side affects. She developed a rash while on Topamax, thus it was replaced by Trileptal. Trileptal is related to Tegretol, and it is an anti-seizure medication, and used for controlling manic symptoms. As she continued to gain weight (eventually weighing 148 pounds), the Zyprexa was gradually reduced. We tried Geodone for a month with no success.

Tiffany has been the most stable on Zyprexa 2.5 mg to 5 mg at night, Wellbrutrin SR 200 mg twice a day, Trileptal 300 mg twice daily, and Prozac 10 mg daily. Her weight has ranged between 125 to 130 pounds. Her mood has stabilized, and she has been free from psychotic symptoms. She enjoys the responsibilities of her job and says her relationships with her husband and son, are better. She attends therapy when needed, and I see her once every two to three months.

As mentioned in the introduction, personality disorders are included in Axis II of the standard five part psychiatric diagnosis. I am always reluctant to diagnosis an Axis II personality disorder until a patient has been initially stabilized with medication and therapy. By definition, personality disorders are life long, and unchanged by medications. Tiffany's destructive behavior patterns, with seemingly no insight into how they affect her life, along with repeated patterns of mood instability, unstable relationships, impulsive and inappropriate anger, recurrent suicidal threats and gestures, self-mutilation, and paranoid ideation confirm the classic symptoms of Borderline Personality Disorder.

Yet, here is the mystery. When Tiffany is appropriately taking her medications and attending therapy, 95% of the Borderline symptoms have vanished. For years, psychoanalysts and psychiatrists argued that personality disorders are deeply rooted in our psyche, self, soul, personality, or whatever word we choose to name who we are at our ground of our being. The rapid improvement in Tiffany's severe symptoms is typical of what I have seen in my clinical practice. This improvement, however, does not mean personal and job stressors cannot quickly tip the delicate equilibrium of her brain's chemistry. Thus, ongoing therapy is essential for Tiffany.

Philosophies, even mythologies, have evolved around psychological schools hardening the view that changes in thought patterns or behavior are either unachievable or possible only through years of therapy. These schools of thoughts flourished when we did not have the criteria to diagnose and the medications and therapies to treat. Thus there is only one model for treatment of mental illness based on science. Consequently, severe mental illness can—and is—being successfully treated through medications, psychotherapy, honesty, vigilance, spiritual faith, caring, and community support.

Tiffany may never be symptom free, but for her to go about her daily responsibilities, maintaining relationships and job, is a small miracle. She is a walking testimony that hope does not merely endure, but prevails.

CHAPTER 5

I Owe a Duty

I owe a duty, where I cannot love.

Brendan Behan

I don't remember much about those times. I didn't know who I was — just a body — no friends. I wasn't afraid to die. I deserved to die. God gave me a life that I was not taking care of. I tried hard to "Give my life back to God." I felt like a bad mother, a bad wife, a bad friend, a bad person, and a bad patient. I felt very guilty over not being able to handle the kids or my own life. You know, typical mother stuff, but way over the edge.

I was indecisive, forgetful, paranoid, anxious, and began hallucinating. I was hopeless. I couldn't look people in the eye. When I went to the doctor's office, I sat on the floor, feeling small and powerless. Most of the time, I stayed in my room writing about myself. We were having marriage problems at the time, and one day I found all my journals in Jeff's filing cabinet. I started shaking, worrying he would use them against me in a divorce, so I burned all of them.

A psychiatrist in Omaha, Nebraska, tried several different medications. Finally, he scheduled electroshock therapy. I had 12 treatments; my husband said they worked temporarily. But nothing really seemed to help. I didn't care what he did to me anymore. I just wanted to die.

Jeff was transferred again, this time to Arizona. He went to work, and I tried to set up housekeeping and get the kids settled. I found a new psychiatrist who tried Buspar, Serzone, Ativan, Ambien, Remeron, and Risperdal. None of them touched the empty despair wilting my soul. Then, my doctor told me that I was not on her managed health care plan and would have to find another psychiatrist.

My new psychiatrist was Dr. Charles; I overdosed twice under his care. His diagnosis was severe depression with psychotic episodes. There were also times when I would suddenly become conscious but had no idea where I was — or how I got there. I am a nurse and have enough experience to know these were dissociative episodes. Then it would happen again. I would "wake up" in the wilderness of Arizona, having no idea how to get home. Sometimes there is a twisted humor in how the mentally ill try to solve their problems. I treated the condition by stuffing my glove compartment with maps of the Southwest.

I became friends with my new neighbor in Arizona. As we talked, one afternoon Bryan told me about his son Greg. He had shot himself in the head a just a few months before we moved. I asked what it was like — having a son who killed himself. He spoke about the love and anger he felt toward his son as well as his own depression, frustration, and guilt. Bryan told me where he found his son and how the police were very judgmental when they interviewed him and his wife. I tried to put myself in Bryan's shoes and imagine what it must have been like — finding his son. I couldn't understand.

I turned and went back to my own house, crawled in the tub with my husband's gun, and held the steel in my mouth. If the gun jerked, it wouldn't miss the easy target. It seemed logical to do it in the tub, so it would be easy to clean.

I clicked back the firing pin as the metallic taste numbed my mouth. Suddenly, one of my children came screaming into the house for something to eat. I put the gun away and went back to my duties. Shortly after, my husband was transferred again; the family packed and moved to North Carolina.

I found a new doctor in Charlotte, and he began trying different drug combinations. He sent me to a psychologist. They both made me sign a contract saying I wouldn't hurt myself. One night I couldn't sleep, so I took more sleeping pills than I should have. Jeff found me non-responsive; he took me to the ER, where they pumped my stomach and admitted me for the night. The psychiatrist called the day I came home and said he wouldn't treat me anymore since I broke the contract. My psychologist said the same thing. Soon, the medications ran out and I stopped seeing anyone. The black hole I had been living in was swallowing me again.

Once, there were days of light. I remember my brother making me climb the Magnolia tree to make sure it was sturdy enough for him to spy on the neighbors; he was such a big chicken.

We lived in a suburban neighborhood full of kids. Mother couldn't have chosen a better house to echo her self. It was a typical '60s split-level, but it had big white columns on the front.

Dad came home from work every night at 5:30. He went to the living room, where he and Mother would have a drink and spend time with each other while the kids were setting the table and getting everything ready.

After dinner, Dad went back to the living room as happy hour drinks changed from beers to scotch and water. Every night it was the same. He passed out on the floor; mother woke him up at midnight and helped him to bed. Thankfully, Dad was a very passive drinker.

My mother was not passive about anything. She was raised in Pennsylvania and told stories of my grandfather beating her. She moved to North Carolina and married my father to get away from him; ever since, she considered herself very Southern. She was an RN who mainly nursed her anger and resentment for having to work.

I remember her double chins that tumbled from her chin to her large belly; she was about five seven and still has dark curly hair. In my mind, she was always strange, different from other mothers. Mother was a very angry woman.

Dad's drinking enraged Mom; while he was putting himself to sleep, or after she put him to bed, she would yell, scream, and beat whoever crossed her path.

God was very real and close those days. I felt He was looking out and protecting me, mostly from my mother. It started when I was five or six; she would hit me with a belt, yardstick, and piece of wood, whatever was close at hand. The strikes smacked my back and head. When I cried, she hit even harder. She seemed to want to beat me hard enough so I would cry.

Mom had a lot of problems. The worst was that she was never wrong. But I have worked through my problems with my mother. Faith has been a big help, knowing it was not my fault. She was just angry.

She told my sister Barb and me how much she hated little girls and loved little boys. We became tomboys, and even though she made us wear dresses, we threw rocks and played army games with the boys. I remember — with neither guilt nor triumph — the time I took a brick and hit a friend; I remember he needed a number of stitches.

We built a tree house next to a neighbor's stable where she kept a mean, stubborn pony.The fort was only a few feet off the ground (which was good since I am afraid of heights). The floor was covered with nails that either missed their mark or never needed to be pounded in the first place. From the bottom, there were hundreds of ugly nails pointing through the floor looking down on you.

Our black miniature poodle Calis was the best friend I ever had. I sat on top of the stairs with her, patting her for hours as she licked away my tears. It was very hard when she died. I was 13 and found out when I came back from a date. Even then, I didn't have a curfew as long as I was on a date.

Mother picked out our clothes, colleges, and jobs. Women were nurses and secretaries and men should be accountants or engineers. I candy-striped at the local hospital not long after Calis died. I brought patients their dinners, cleaned their rooms, took care of whatever they needed — basically it was doing the same things I was doing at home, but the patients said thank you.

At 15, I was an aide at Duke Hospital. The RNs knew I wanted to be a nurse, so they let me touch the patients. There was one middle-aged woman who had abdominal surgery; they left the incision unsutured, and each day I would help open the wound, clean her belly, and repack it with gauze.

Today, I work on a floor that is a mix of cancer and post-operative patients. It is quiet; I spend most of the time teaching them how to go home. I teach them what they should be doing for themselves. I sit with them and try to make them feel comfortable. I do what I'm told.

I always have, even when Mom ridiculed and pitted Barb and me against each other.Mother picked swimming to be the sport for her five children. Barbara was a fine swimmer with a grace in her stroke that was beautiful to watch. She swam in the Junior Olympics one year. The only times Barb ever heard kind words, or felt support from our parents, was for her swimming.

Barb has always been a computer person, skinny, and a typical anorexic. When attacked, I would curl in, talk to the dog or rabbit; Barb would fight. She went through a period of not having a job for almost two years. Ignoring everyone's advice, she stayed in New York, spending all her savings until she finally found a position. She did stay with us in Chicago when Jeff and I were first married (rent-free). She came home from work, staying in her room the rest of the time, isolating herself from the world. Every once in a while, I could get her to watch a TV show with me.

Today, Barbara lives alone with her daughter in New York. Like every mother, she thinks her daughter is the smartest child in the world. Whenever she worries about Morgan, she calls me. I am like a husband to her in that I am her best friend. We talk for at least 45 minutes. I only say a few words as every subject is gently turned toward her. I don't confront Barb or give advice, because she does the exact opposite of what anyone tells her to do.

When Barb was a senior at Duke, she overdosed on sleeping pills and was hospitalized. She wouldn't let our parents see her. Her therapists said she needed a safe person to talk to. I was and am that person.

She needs help, and I am supposed to give it.

Since Barb was the best in swimming, I was told that I was not trying. Both of us were called ugly because our younger sister Carol is beautiful. She is tall, leggy, and has dark blond hair. She got average grades in high and loved attention from the boys. Today, she lives in a nice house in Raleigh, a very upscale neighborhood inside the beltway. She hangs out at the country club and their beach house. Her first daughter, Erin, is Carol's splitting image; both are competitive, always wanting to keep up with friends. You cannot have deep conversation with her; she loves to gossip and chatter with her girlfriends.

I would not consider Carol a friend. She always argues and criticizes, but she is a good source for information. If I want to know if my parents enjoyed a visit to my home, I call Carol. She knows every detail, and always remembers at least one negative comment my parents reported. She is self-centered but having a great time.

And if she is happy, then I am happy for her.

My brother Sherwood was the first child, born two years before me. He loved his name and said it was "The best name in the world!" Every time we had a child, he called from whatever city he was currently living in and said I should name the new baby Sherwood. He worked in a high stress job, always moving. He ended in Atlanta, where he developed lymphoma. The last few months, he came home to Durham, where he died at 42.

Sherwood married his mother. Leigh loves to boss and command. They met when she was at a girl's school and he was at NC State. Leigh and I still talk on the phone, its easy; all I have to say is "Yea, yea" between subjects.

My youngest brother is Doug. He really had a hard time. Our mother constantly let Barb and me know how awful we were and how we were ruining her life. Anything bad that happened was our fault. We went to school covered with bruises. No one ever asked. We never spoke to anyone about the abuse; it was too embarrassing.

Then in seventh grade, somehow I ended up on the cheerleading squad. I was instantly popular. However, there was such a space between how my new friends treated me and what went on at home that I began to slip between that distance, unsure of my worth and who I was.

I went to a Christian group called Young Life in tenth grade. My parents did not approve of the college kids leading the group. So I would sneak out the sliding door and walk three blocks to the meetings. It was there I accepted Jesus Christ and learned there were people in the world who were in even worse shape than I was. I began to think of others and not myself all the time.

I took a job at the mall when I was 16.

One weekend, my parents went out of town with the younger kids, leaving my older brother and me at home. It was a Saturday night; I came home from work and found my brother drinking beer and playing cards with three friends. I went to bed.

My brother eventually passed out; his three friends came downstairs and found me. They held me down and took turns raping me — one after the other. I felt all the usual feelings: dirty, guilty, thinking I caused it to happen, that it was my fault. I couldn't scrub my body hard enough to get off the filth. I cried alone for weeks but not in front of anyone. I never told a person until the depression came.

In high school, my mother would not let me go out with a group of girls. She thought they were just trying to get picked up. However, it was all right for me to date boys. So, as often as possible, I staged a date with a buddy to get out of the house and away from Mother. I became active in school: cheerleading, pep club, yearbook staff, student council, and service clubs, anything to get out of the house. I never received a B, only straight A's.

Then the varsity football coach asked me to meet him to talk about something he needed help with. When I met him after school, he took me to the health room and raped me. I stayed out of school for three days with a "stomach virus" until I could find enough courage to go back.

The only adult I ever loved was my grandmother. Grammy was a wonderful Southern lady from another world, a place of tradition where the word "home" was synonymous with love.

She raised my father as a single mother before there was a term to define that sadness. She had a quick mind and knew that manners were a way for different generations to talk to each other. She spoke proper English with a soft, lyrical, Southern tone. Quick to correct our grammar, she taught me to be a lady and hold my head high, even when I felt like crawling under a rock. Grammy was not allowed in our house because Mother did not like her. We were not to visit or call. But I would sneak over and see her as often as possible.

At 92, she was still strong and kind, living alone in her own home. A 13-year-old boy broke into her house for her car keys. When she refused, he killed her, and then chopped her body into little pieces.

It was a horrific, sickening time. I went to the trial. I listened to that boy's story of how bad his life had been. I cried for him. And I felt cold, pure anger for the first time in my life. He went to juvenile detention and was released five years later when he turned 18.

The darkness began to take over me when I decided to attend Chapel Hill. Since both my parents graduated from Duke, the Tar Heels were already the enemy in our house. The first few months at school, I fell in love with a sweet boy, but he was Italian Catholic and my parents said I couldn't date him. Mom called Tony and told him to "stay with his own kind."

I read in the Bible that you should honor your mother and father, so we broke up, and I broke apart. I started partying -- our drink was Seven and Sevens, and they never stopped. The only thing I took seriously was the elderly outpatient I was helping through a social work class. I drove her to the doctor, gave her money for groceries, but I never wrote down my case notes. The professor was furious that I was crossing boundaries I didn't know existed. I failed the class and quit school my freshman year.

I called the nursing school at the University of North Carolina, Charlotte and told the dean of the nursing school that I had dropped out of school.Her response was kind; she said, "Sometimes it is just not the right time; why don't you come to Charlotte for a year and see how it goes." I met Jeff in Charlotte. He was the president of two Christian groups on campus. The first time I saw him, I thought he was the loudest, most obnoxious person I ever met. But we became good friends. He is the person everyone loved, a heart of gold, and so honestly nice that some people thought it was a façade.

He has always been a leader and seemed to have everything under control. I was so happy when we married. Jeff was a wonderful man with a strong faith; he had dreams for a family. Raised in a stable loving home, he was a positive thinker, proud of himself and his accomplishments. He also had a good job, was cute, and kind. He truly loved me even though I felt so unlovable. Jeff honestly wanted to make me happy. Soon after we married, I realized a darker side as Jeff's control became dominating. Before our children were born, and when we had time together, he told me which dresses I could buy. He is a big spender and very generous; it was a control issue. He wanted to dress me up into something I wasn't. I should have told Jeff to leave me alone on personal decisions.

We bought a station wagon and eagerly awaited the arrival of children. I had been in nursing school for several years and had experience in surgery, pediatrics, intensive care, and recovery. I was eager to tackle motherhood. I got pregnant right away. But the day we moved from North Carolina to Chicago, I had a miscarriage. I was devastated. When I called my mother to tell her, she said it was a good thing because Sherwood should have the first grandchild.

Jeff Adam (named for his father) was born two years latter. He was wonderful. In the Southern tradition, we called him by his middle name. Adam, it means a gift from God. His sister Anne Marian, "Anne," was named after her great-grandmothers. There was difficulty with the pregnancy and I was in and out of the hospital for several months. The pressure began to wear.

Each pregnancy and child came with increasing stress. James Alexander ("Alex") was born very early. He was in intensive care for several weeks waiting for surgery. It was a time of prayers and tears. I found him blue one day, and after several tests, it was diagnosed that his heart would occasionally just stop beating. His breathing was even worse, stopping 50 to 60 times a day. His body began to collapse after surgery, and he was placed on a respirator. The doctor said to call the family, as Alex would not make it through the night. Miraculously, he survived until morning, then the next day, and the day after. He had breathing and heart problems for two years. Our fourth child, Melissa Ashley ("Ashley") was born in Florida with the same condition as Alex. It was another year of monitors and heart-stopping nights.

We moved to Atlanta for seven months, then to Nebraska where Sherwood Allan was born. I finally named a child Sherwood, but we call him "Allan." I named him after a high school boyfriend, a sweet guy with a heart of gold. Allan had the same heart and breathing condition as his siblings; when he got well enough to get off the monitors and oxygen, I finally had time to think about myself. It struck me that I had five children, just like my mother. I wanted to raise my family without the yelling, in a loving and kind home. But I worried if I could do any better than Mom.

Then the bottom fell out. There was just too much sadness. It was during this time that both my younger brother and Barb tried to commit suicide. It was also when my aunt and older brother died of cancer, and mother had surgery for an abdominal malignancy.

I fell apart. I felt neglected by Jeff, who was constantly working. He was so busy and stressed that he came home complaining about the house being a mess, dinner not being ready, or the children not behaving. He would bark orders at the children and me, and if the kids didn't comply, he would yell and threaten to spank them. He did a lot of yelling and screaming back then. His unhinged anger reminded me of my mother.

I spent 14 years having five children and five miscarriages. Jeff was a workaholic, traveled all week, and went to the office on weekends. He was afraid to help with the little ones on monitors and did not become close to any of our children.He never learned CPR, so I could not leave him with the babies; he was afraid they would die.

Yet Jeff cared. I have always loved horses. During a particularly down time he gave me Zeke. He was very friendly and let the children pat him on the nose. He was calm as could be, but he had a rough canter. Ninety percent of the time I would talk to him in the pasture. He was my one friend who would listen. I would tell him about what the children were going through and my latest stress; he just stood there and listened.

Yet the darkness grew. I couldn't focus; was tired but could never sleep, eat, or work up enough energy to take care of my children or the house. I lost interest in everything that ever mattered. Even though I was in awful shape, I refused to see the doctor. I became dehydrated from not eating. Then paranoia set in as I thought Jeff was going to beat me. I finally curled up on the bed and spent the day crying. My friend called a doctor, who sent a home health nurse that day to start IVs. He told my friend what to do if things got any worse.

I finally felt a little better, but when my friend went home, I took an overdose of pills. It was the first of eight times I tried to kill myself. Somehow, someone would always find me and take me to the hospital and I would be in the ER having my stomach pumped. The neighbors worked together to make sure someone checked on me daily.

I felt so guilty because I was not able to handle my children or even my own life. I was indecisive, forgetful, hopeless, paranoid, anxious, and began hallucinating. I couldn't look people in the eye.

We moved from Nebraska to Arizona and I began the ECT treatments. The last time I tried to take my life was with the gun. I wasn't trying; I wanted it to happen. The only thing that stopped me was Alex coming in the house screaming for something to eat. The only thing I felt more than the pain and loneliness was my duty to my children.

Looking back, few things make sense. During the worst times, I lay in bed, but my heart beat so fast I literally couldn't count my pulse. All I wanted to do was die, but at the same time I was terrified that each of us are given so many heartbeats in a lifetime and I was racing through

We moved again, this time to Charlotte. After my therapist and psychiatrist refused to treat me, I decided to see a Christian counselor. I found a church with a behavioral clinic. The director met with me several times and knew I need more help than he could give; he sent me to Dr. Sethi. I began personal counseling, and Jeff and I began marriage counseling.

The nights passed slowly. It took two years of intense counseling and many medication adjustments before I could see the morning star.

Am I happy? Sometimes. Better yet, there is stability. That horrible feeling, that the ground is opening to swallow me in utter blackness, has faded.

After I got involved in church, in typical fashion, Jeff jumped back under full steam. He heads a Bible study and will probably be running the church soon. Things are not perfect with us, but I know he loves me, and he has always tried to give me the one thing no person can give another — happiness. Is there a perfect marriage where both people are content? I don't think so. That is why we make pledges that carry us through the hard times.

Was my sickness caused by bad genetics or from my troubled family? Probably both. Is my pain anyone's fault? Of course, not. I have not had an easy life, but there are others who have suffered far more than I have without developing a mental illness. One thing the pain has taught me is that life is precious beyond the words to tell. It is neither ours to give or take, but to cherish. I am learning how to receive as much as I give, to love – well, at least appreciate—myself. There is still pain to heal and so much to change.

Psychiatric Assessment

The thought of suicide is a great source of comfort: with it a calm passage is to be made across many a bad night.

Friedrich Nietzsche

A suicide kills two people, Maggie, that's what it's for!

Arthur Miller

Never the sentimentalist, the German philosopher Nietzsche saw life as a war without mercy; meant to be won by the strong. As so many before and after, Nietzsche viewed suicide as an escape for the weak. And of course, it often devastates those who are left to wonder if the death could have been prevented. Suicide is the cruelest of afflictions because the victim is often blamed for his or her death. Like Dante, we reserve a special place in hell for suicides, believing they chose to speak only through their blood.

Perhaps a better wisdom is gained from the writer and physician Walker Percy who said to beware of any science or religion that takes the mystery out of what it means to live and die and be a human being. There is a fine line between a martyr and a suicide, and sometimes only a twist of circumstances separating the artist from the creative genius who can no longer bear the pain. Percy said that most successful writers are unsuccessful suicides—those who have peered into the abyss, stopped, and turned toward home to write about it. Many who have attempted suicide later say that, at the time, they truly believed the world—and their closest friends and family—would have been better off without them.

We, who live among and treat those who think about taking their own lives, must avoid cut and dried answers to this terrible mystery, whether we respond with science or philosophy.What we do know is that among all psychiatric illnesses, depression caries the highest risk for suicide, followed by alcohol and other substance abuse. The combination of depression and alcohol is extremely dangerous.

At every session, I evaluate all my patients who may have suicidal intentions with the blunt question, "Have you felt any suicidal thoughts, and if so, have you made any specific plans to take your life."

On a scale of one to ten, with one being the worst and ten being none, Carrie rated her suicidal thoughts at a ten. However, with her history of multiple hospitalizations and numerous suicide attempts, Carrie was a high-risk patient. She came to my office because her most recent psychiatrist and therapist terminated their treatments because she violated their "No Harm" contract. These contracts are additionally helpful to patients to see that others really do care if they live or die. For patients like Carrie, their sense of obligation can be made tangible by signing a pledge. During her first appointment, Carrie and I made a verbal "No Harm" contract. She promised not to hurt herself, and if she had overwhelming thoughts of suicide, pledged she would call

911, go to the nearest emergency room, call her therapist, friend, or my office as well as schedule an early appointment.

However, as Carrie and I made this verbal covenant, I was also answering my own moral questions. "Should I accept this patient, and treat her with the best of my clinical abilities, or should I protect myself from a potential malpractice suit?" One of the "hidden" concerns behind "No Harm" covenants is that caregivers are often attempting to protect themselves from litigation. Under these circumstances, I must answer the critical ethical question of whether I should treat the patient or be cowered by the threat of a law suit. In most cases, I have chosen the former. I feel strongly that among physicians, and other health-care workers, psychiatrists are the best qualified to treat these patients.

In the end, we all must remember that we are flawed human beings. I often remind myself, and sometimes tell my patients of those people who had the best possible care available, and still took their own lives. Vince Foster, a powerful White House legal counsel, and a trusted friend of First Lady and President Clinton, committed suicide. Despite his connections and resources, he did not seek help from the severe depression that took his life.

Several years ago, a respected psychiatrist in Charlotte who worked with 10 other psychiatrists in an established group practice, committed suicide with carbon monoxide poisoning. When I was an Associate Professor with the Oncology Research Center at the Bowman Gray School of Medicine of Wake Forest University in Winston-Salem, North Carolina, a close friend and colleague took his own life. John's wife is a pediatrician, and he was a Ph.D., and an M.D. research oncologist. Yet, despite access to the best psychiatric and medical care, they could not help themselves. If a person is determined to commit suicide, as with my colleagues, Drs. Caudel and Stewart, even the best psychiatric care, or numerous hospitalizations, cannot save them. Do cardiologists and oncologists refuse to treat their patients who relapse into the lifestyles that contributed to their illnesses—of course not? Psychiatrists, like all people who attempt to help others, must, as the Spanish writer Ortega said, take a look at the storm about them with a "ruthless, tragic glance," and then do their very best.

When Carrie came into my office she was seeing a Christian, faith-based counselor as well as a marriage therapist. She was taking Celexa 40 mg daily, Ritalin 20 mg in the morning, and Ambien 20 mg at night for sleep. She also took Lorazepam 1 mg as needed for anxiety. She tried Buspar 10 mg, three times a day, but discontinued from the side effects of feeling groggy and sleepy.

Her presenting symptoms were: sleeplessness, barely functioning at home with her five children, feeling very depressed with low self-esteem, and a loss of appetite with a corresponding weight loss. While Carrie said she had not made any specific plans to hurt herself, she had been struggling with suicidal thoughts for at least four years, and firearms had been taken out of the house.

Carrie said she had no symptoms of mania, eating disorders, explosive rages; or symptoms of anxiety, panic, or obsessive-compulsive (e.g. excessive cleaning, repeatedly checking doors or locks, placing items in order, mental obsession, and rituals) disorders. She described a mild paranoia concerning other people, but was not hearing voices or experiencing visual hallucinations. She drinks wine socially, but had no history of alcohol, drug, cigarette, caffeine, or over-the-counter medication abuse. She was taking Pepcid for gastric reflux and birth control pills.

On a scale of one to ten, ten being the best and one being the worst, Carrie described her overall functioning at three, relationships with her children three to four and two with her husband, and social settings as a two to three. On the same scale, ten having no psychiatric symptoms and one being the worst, she described her depression at two, anxiety four, and suicidal thoughts ten.

Carrie was a full time home maker, and taking care of her five children between the ages of 5 to 14. Two of the children had depression, and they were being treated by a child psychiatrist.

She began seeking professional help for her depression in Omaha five years before her most recent move to Charlotte, NC. She was treated with numerous medications such as Prozac, Paxil, Wellbutrin, Remeron, Serzone, Effexor, Ativan, Xanax, Buspar, Chloral Hydrate, Ambien, Zyprexa, Risperdal, Ritalin, and Depakote. She was hospitalized more than six times in Nebraska where she received 12 electroshock treatments and had been hospitalized several times in Arizona.She stated her diagnosis was Major Depression, Passive-aggressive, and Borderline Personality Disorders.

Carrie was born and raised in Durham, NC. Her mother was very strict and controlling. She was raped at the age of 16 by friends of her brother and then again in high school and college at the age of 17 and 18. Her parents are in their early seventies and retired. They live in Pinehurst, NC. Her father used to drink heavily, and her grandmother was also alcoholic. She was brutally murdered at the age of 92 by a 13 year old boy in the neighborhood. Carrie has two brothers and two sisters. One brother died of cancer, and the other has depression. Also one of her sisters has depression, and she has been hospitalized.

Carrie went to University of North Carolina for her BS in Nursing. She met her husband there. She has been married for 18 years to Jeff, and they have five children ranging from 5 to 14 years. Two of her children suffer from depression. Jeff is of same age as Carrie, and he is Vice President of Sales of a national food company. He travels a lot on his job. His parents also live in Pinehurst, NC. Carrie stopped working 14 years ago when her son was born. She is a full time mother and wife. The family moved to Charlotte from Arizona six moths ago. They are renting an apartment while their 5,000 square feet house is being built.

Carrie said she felt stressed from her recent move, living in an apartment, marital problems made worse by her husband's frequent travel, her illness, and her responsibility for her children. She feels support from her children, therapist and neighbor. Her strength includes having a good physical health, a good profession, being attractive, having no financial problems and a supportive husband.

As a nurse, she gave me a good history of her medical psychiatric treatments. She also recalled her early family traumas and serious afflictions during childhood and adolescence. She was friendly and made good eye contact, though her mood was clearly very depressed. She was very withdrawn, yet she was alert and well oriented to time, place, and person. Her memory and thoughts were clear. She spoke softly. Her speech was linear and goal oriented, and she was well dressed in casual clothes.

Based on these finding, my diagnosis was that Carrie suffered from a chronic and recurrent Major Depressive Disorder. However, I was not sure of her Borderline and Passive Aggressive Personality Disorders traits.

Despite taking a high dose of Ambien, Carrie was not sleeping well. Therefore, I substituted Ambien with Trazodone. Further, she was eating little and losing weight, so I prescribed Remeron, which also helps to sleep better and it improves appetite.

Trazodone was developed as an antidepressant in mid eighties, a few years earlier than Prozac. It is strongly sedating and used clinically as a sleeping agent. Serzone is chemically related to Trazodone, but is a stronger antidepressant and less sedating.

Trazodone, also called Desyrel, has one serious and rather unusual side effect in men. In rare instances, it causes males to have continued erections after intercourse and masturbation. This condition must be treated in an emergency room, or the patient may lose his penis. While the side effect occurs one in 40,000 patients, we generally warn all male patients.

Carrie was continued on her Celexa and Ritalin, and instructed to take Ambien only when needed. I asked her to bring a list detailing the types and amounts of all her medications at home. As she had seen so many psychiatrists, I asked her to write her goals and expectations. A return appointment was made within seven to ten days.

When she came for her next session in seven days, Carrie was taking Celexa 40 mg, Remeron 15 mg, and Trazodone 50 mg at night. She had stopped the Ritalin on her own. Her sleep was improving to four to six sustained hours at night, but she was still feeling slightly groggy for the first two to three hours in the morning. Carrie's appetite was improving, and she had a good weekend talking with her husband.

She brought a list of her medications. She was going out of the house every day, and was earnestly trying to improve. Her thoughts of suicide were subsiding, and she had written her goals and was feeling optimistic they could be achieved. Since she was still feeling depressed and anxious, I increased her Remeron to 30 mg and decreased the Trazodone to 25 mg to see if it would reduce her morning grogginess. I also prescribed Ativan to be taken for anxiety as needed.

During her third visit ten days later, Carrie said she was eating better and her depression was lifting slightly. She was not crying as much, but Carrie felt overwhelmed with their move, taking care of her five children with their many games and parties, and was tiring easily. Further, she reported some spotting and cramps and suspected fibroid tumor. She was concerned of a recent hair loss and increasing lethargic feelings. Carrie said she was not having any suicidal thoughts. In response to these effects, I discontinued her Remeron, increased the Trazodone to 100 mg at night for sleep, and started her on Wellbutrin, which is a stimulating antidepressant. It helps to reduce tiredness, and improve concentration and focus.

Carrie continued to feel stressed by her need for a hysterectomy due to the fibroids. Her 11-year-old son was advised to have brain surgery for a soccer accident, and her insurance company was stalling on approving the necessary surgery. In addition, Carrie's husband was traveling five days a week on business. She continued to be tearful and tired, but assured me she was not having any suicidal thoughts. As she was tolerating Wellbutrin 75 mg twice daily without side effects, its dose was gradually increased to 200 mg twice daily. Trazodone was also increased to 200 mg for continual improvement in her sleep patterns.

After a few months, Carrie's condition began to deteriorate. Her environmental and physical stressors were simply overwhelming. Within a relatively brief period, Carrie had: laparoscopic surgery for fibroids, was helping one son recover from brain surgery while two others were being treated for depression, and she had wrecked both family cars in the same month. Further, her insurance company stopped payments for her psychiatric treatment as she had already used her yearly number of mental health sessions. All these stressors deepened her depression and she began having visual hallucinations of little men in the grocery store, and saw items moving around her home as well as hearing the TV speak to her. Her suicidal thoughts returned, but she denied formulating any specific plans. In view of these new symptoms, I added the antipsychotic medication Risperdal to her list of medications, and scheduled an appointment every one to two weeks. I also asked Carrie to bring her husband to the next visit and count all the pills at home.

At this time, I revised her diagnosis from Major Depressive Disorder, severe, recurrent to Major Depressive Disorder, severe, recurrent, with psychotic features.

I educated Jeff about the complexities of Carrie's illness and the rationale of diagnosis and treatment. Further, he was advised that she must go to the hospital should her suicide thoughts become out of control, and also advised about the procedure for involuntary commitment. I further warned them that I shall be obliged to dismiss her from the practice as the previous psychiatrist did should she fail to go to the hospital prior to overdosing or hurting herself. They were further cautioned about her driving. At this point, I increased her dose of Trazodone to 400 mg and Risperdal gradually from 1 mg to 3 mg at night.

Within two weeks Carrie started to improve. She came with her dog to the office. She was smiling a little, and she weighed a healthy 137 pounds. Jeff was coming home every night. Her sister from Raleigh had come to help. She was getting up early, and doing all chores. Her suicidal thoughts were starting to subside, but not gone completely. Visual hallucinations were better. She was still hearing voices from the TV, and thus stopped watching. In view of this I increased her Risperdal to 4.5 mg, and she continued on Celexa 40 mg, Wellbutrin SR 200 mg twice daily, and Trazodone 200 mg at night.

At this session within two weeks, Carrie reported milky discharge from her breasts. Her overall functioning at home was better. She had gone to the church after 3 months for the first time, and did not feel paranoid. She was not hearing voices and had no hallucinations. She was still not watching TV, although she was not getting any special messages. Her suicidal thoughts continued, but not intensely. She was smiling more. I reduced her Risperdal to 3 mg, and recommended a CT scan of the head to rule out any tumor of the pituitary. Carrie told me that she had a similar experience in Nebraska, and at that time her CT and MRI scans of the head were negative.

At her next session in three weeks, Carrie came with Jeff. She was making satisfactory progress. She was feeling more positive, finishing her work at home, attending the children's activities, and had started going to the gym. She was also attending church and Bible studies. Carrie was joking more; she and Jeff were feeling optimistic about their future and visibly cherished each other. The hallucinations and suicidal thoughts were gone. Carrie continued to be anxious that she was sleeping too much. In response, I reduced the Trazodone dosage and scheduled an appointment in five weeks.

At this next visit, she reported having a good Christmas and New Year. She went to parties with Jeff and had a good time. She turned 43, and had a birthday party at home. She continued going to church and attending Bible studies. She complained of sleeping a lot, and discharge from her breasts coming back. She said she would like to discontinue the Risperdal. I reduced the Trazodone to 50 mg and Risperdal to 2 mg.

Within six weeks of reducing the Risperdal, Carrie began to see spiders, hear strange noises in the house as well as the alarm clock ringing all the time. She looked for noises everywhere in the home. She began to feel irritable, complained about the children's misbehavior, and Jeff's inattention. Jeff and Carrie were also concerned about one of their sons who was caught by the police stealing road signs. In addition, she was understandably angry with her insurance company for not paying her past four visits. She denied stopping her medication.

We discussed her past history of stopping medications and subsequent return of her symptoms, and of how well she had done a few months ago. She said she had not reduced her medications. Her dosage of Risperdal was increased to 3 mg, and she was reminded of our "No Harm" contract. I decided to increase the frequency of her sessions.

It was spring, and Carrie recalled that she had been hospitalized at this same time during the past several years. This may appear strange, but some individuals are especially sensitive to psychiatric symptoms during a certain season of the year. In my practice, I have noted deterioration of symptoms even leading to hospitalizations with a certain periodicity. It is well known that increase in stressors or the anniversary of certain events can certainly affect the course of illness. It is puzzling sometimes, when without any undue stressors, some chronic patients exhibit recurrence of symptoms with a certain frequency. Thus it becomes critical to follow theses patients regularly on an ongoing basis.

Carrie started to improve by the end of April. She resumed all her social, church and family responsibilities. She went through a hysterectomy by the middle of May, and was hospitalized for 3 days. Jeff took some time off from work to take care of her and the children. They went to Richmond, VA to visit family. Summer went smoothly without any problems. She had a new Therapist, and continued with marital therapy. She got a maid to help with house chores. She gained enough confidence and went back to complete her refresher courses in Nursing at UNC-Charlotte.

Christmas is a rough season for many. Carrie arranged a party for 50 people at her home, and did well. Despite the usual stressors of children, season, and mother-in-law coming to visit, she did not relapse. She felt confident to reduce Risperdal to 2 mg and Trazodone from 100 mg to 75 mg. She made all A's in her course work, and started clinical rotations at the Carolina Medical Center. I continued to see her once a month.

By the first week in April, Carrie was strongly urged by her therapist to see me on an emergency basis. Her mood was depressed, and she was not eating and feeling tired. Suicidal thoughts were beginning to return. There were contributing environmental stressors. She had recently seen her dog killed by a passing car. She was working on the Oncology floor, caring for many dying patients, and her supportive neighbor had been away for a week. Whether it was these factors or Carrie's vulnerability to spring weather (or the collective pressure of all these factors) that prompted her relapse is difficult to assess. In response, I increased her Risperdal to 3 mg and Celexa to 60 mg per day; the other medications were kept at the same dosage.

Despite these pharmacological changes, Carrie's mood was not lifting. She had graduated with all A's, Jeff took her to the Kentucky Derby, the family got a new dog, but Carries continued to be severely depressed. She felt tired and lethargic and did not wish to switch from Celexa to Effexor as the latter had caused a "bad reaction."

When severely depressed patients do not respond well to antidepressants, at their highest dosages, I have had good success with stimulants such as Dexedrine and Ritalin. Since Carrie had no history of substance abuse, I prescribed Dextrastat, also known as Dextroamphetamine. As this and other stimulants can be addictive, I would not have been comfortable prescribing this medication to a patient with a history of substance abuse. In less than two weeks, Carrie said the new medication at 15 mg twice daily changed her mood from "night into day." She had more energy and was exercising daily at the YMCA. She enjoyed a recent vacation to Charleston with her family and was looking forward to a new nursing position. She was not suffering any delusions and had no side affects from the new medications.

Carrie continued to improve and commented that she "had not felt this well in years." She became far more active, handling her job, children, and social interactions quite well. It was frustrating for both of us when Carrie's insurance company denied coverage for the Dextroamphetamine, saying that she had no history of attention deficit disorder. I called the insurance company and spoke with their staff pharmacist who blankly said coverage was denied because it did not follow the company guidelines. I had my own brief explosive moment as I told the pharmacist this prescription was likely saving her company tens of thousands of dollars from a potential hospitalization. Finally, this medication was approved for six-week intervals, as long as a nurse from our office called for prior approval.Out of shear frustration in not being able to treat a patient with my best medical judgment, I finally spoke with the insurance company's Medical Director, who approved the Dexedrine for six months at a time.

Carrie went through a rough Spring. With reluctance she went back to full dosages of medications. Jeff got a big promotion at his job of being national sales manager, and he need not travel as much. But he still leaves the house at 5:30 AM and comes back at 8 PM. Carrie is working one day a week. She is exercising again and socializing at church functions. She has been very scared of war in Iraq. She is happy with her family. She is currently taking Risperdal 2 mg, Wellbutrin SR 200 mg twice daily, Celexa 60 mg, Trazodone 100 to 150 mg, Dextroamphetamine 10 mg twice daily, and Ambien 10 mg as needed.

One of the tragedies in managed health care is this trend to take responsibility and authority away from physicians. Many health care workers, especially those who treat the mentally ill, are becoming increasing frustrated as managed care prevents them from doing what they know is medically best for the patient. Since it involves the mystery of what it means to be a person, medicine remains an art as much as it is a science. As such, black and white answers, to most medical situations, especially psychiatric ones, are rarely helpful.

Cancer, heart disease, AIDS, and other complex illnesses are often treated by numerous medications and complex therapies. It is difficult for many patients to manage a disease requiring multiple pills to be taken throughout the day. This is particularly true in psychiatry where mental health patients suffer the additional stigma of a society that gives the message that "only really crazy people have to see a psychiatrist." Taking numerous medications at the proper time is a major challenge in compliance. I try to help by educating my patients about their diagnosis and the rational for the medications and their side effects. Like many who suffer a serious and lifelong illness, Carrie still does not like to take medications. If there were only one or two pills, she might not mind, but six pills is a lot. Carrie has taken herself off the Risperdal several times only to find her psychotic and depressive symptoms returning. The vast majority of mental illnesses are treatable, but physicians, insurance companies, and patients must realize that treatment sometimes takes a lifetime of diligent management. Perhaps the next generation of medications may make this easier.

It is a tragedy that many insurance companies judge the severity of mental illness based upon the number of medications that a patient is taking, and they are charging higher premiums with more numbers of psychotropic medications. This is nonsense, and blatant discrimination against psychiatric illnesses which are biologically based, and need pharmacological treatment. Through carve out and other maneuvering the insurance companies have put a life-long cap in treatment of psychiatric illnesses. I sincerely hope that with better education from these true life stories, the patients and politicians would demand that there be parity between the physical and mental illnesses, as their origins are the same based in chemical differences between the normal and the abnormal.

CHAPTER 6

Beauty Crieth

Dusty, cobweb-covered, maimed, and set at naught,
Beauty crieth in an attic, and no man regardeth
Samuel Butler

Memories of my grandfather are of a thin man with a walking cane. His dog Nippy by his side, and the patch he always wore on his nose.

He still walks through my memory to the family's general store in Stony Point. It's made of native rock. Watermelons were stacked on the front porch. He bought me ice cream, Popsicles, and penny candy from the bins inside. Mary Janes were my favorite — chewy peanut butter candy wrapped in yellow paper — peppermint balls, and peanut butter and cheese crackers. There were wooden barrels full of dried pinto beans and a pot-bellied stove where the farmers talked about the weather and the prices of cotton and tobacco. I can still smell the huge hoops of sharp cheddar. Uncle Ike and Buddy were there a lot and eventually ran the store. Friends from church would stop by; it was the fellowship hall with the same door for family and friends.

The family often spoke of my grandmother, praising her disciplined routine, excellent manners, and the way she always had a nice thing to say about others. As the mother of 11 aunts and uncles, grandmother to countless cousins, everyone knew her and how she died. It wasn't a secret; but it was never told — just there — balancing on the edge of awareness.

She was in the midst of yet another wave of depression, an illness that pounded her all her life. Blind from diabetes, the disease was slowly killing, a piece at a time.

One morning, my grandfather left especially early to open the store. No one else was at home as she reached under her mattress and held her husband's shotgun to her heart. She took her life from us when I was 18 months old. I was living with Aunt Sophie while my mother was having back surgery.

Mom inherited Grandmother's red hair and depression but not her mild nature. There was always a person nearby to trigger her anger. She rose early in the morning for 26 years and left for the mill where she worked as a manager. Every day, I fixed her hair the identical way before she went to work. I fussed, braided, pinned the curls back, tying a ribbon around the back. I never did it well enough to suit --"You're not fixing it right!"

Father was her mirror opposite — good looking, thin, handsome, liked by the women, friendly, and utterly irresponsible. He made you feel good about yourself with a sincere compliment for all the ladies. My aunts loved him. Dad was also a terrible alcoholic. Well, actually, he was quite good at it. Too tight to walk, he would drive all night on country roads and never had an accident. I don't know how he ever made it home. He went to a dry-out center once but ended up in the same shape. He was forever in trouble, writing bad checks or something else. Mom asked us, "Why does he do that?" I remember a time when she was very dependant on a prescription called Miltown. She was really hooked; she stared at us like a Zombie from another world. There were so many things I didn't understand.

Dad felt the weight of his failures. He loved Mother, really loved her, but he never stopped drinking, never *wanted* to stop. Mother worked and stayed at home. Dad drank and stayed away.Scared and depressed, Mom brought order to her world by domineering everyone in it. I quietly rebelled.

She would tell me to clean up the house. Each day, I began a hopeless cleaning frenzy exactly at 3 o'clock — dusting, vacuuming, making the bed, doing the dishes -- knowing I'd never finish in time. There was always something left undone when she walked in the door at 4:30.

Mom loved my brother Jimmy. He was six years older, and I remember him mainly by his absence. Like Dad, he was handsome, had a crew cut, and lots of girls. He was a neat dresser, polishing his black and white oxfords and penny loafers. As a child, Jimmy molded clay football players. He made a complete set for every team in the South, treasuring them in cigar boxes one of our uncles gave him.

He was the ideal son; Mom loved him to death. When he came home on leave from the Marines, there were huge platters of fried chicken for Jimmy and his friends. But when he returned from Vietnam and married, he never came home again. Years later, I called when Dad was dying and told him I couldn't do everything by myself. Jimmy said, "I will help you, but I will never come back to North Carolina." We didn't talk about it, but I understood. Mother would not have tolerated the attention of another woman; she would have broken his marriage. When Jimmy was in the room, she demanded his full, undivided love. Looking back, it is strange that Mother's unconditional anger tied me to home while her jealous love drove Jimmy away.

In their mess of a gene pool, my parents gave me the one thing every girl wants, perhaps even more than love; they gave me beauty — sheer physical good looks. It was as surrounding and present as the poverty of our home. At school, it made me happy. I was the head cheerleader, the school princess. After graduation, I went to a small business school for a year. My parents were struggling financially and really couldn't afford to send me. I was an average student, more interested in boys and my social life than an education.

So, I dropped out of college and took a job as a receptionist for a large oil company. I loved the job and was crowned their Queen at the annual ball and later featured in some advertising. Life seemed to be so good: I had a great job, a nice boyfriend, and was second runner-up in the North Carolina Miss Universe contest. I was trying to make a life of my own, distant from my rocky past. I even enjoyed volunteering for the Red Cross at a local hospital. I had no idea what was ahead for me, but I was having a good time.

I started dating my boyfriend in high school. He seemed to have all the good things I cherished in my father. He was good looking, well-liked, and adored by the girls. But when he was transferred to Birmingham, my world began to crumble.

Our relationship was not always smooth.He loved women, and they were terribly attracted to him. I knew if I didn't do something that I would lose him. So, I left my job and family and moved to Alabama. The toughest part was telling Mom; she despised Edmond. I knew it was a choice she could never reconcile.

Despite Mom's bitterness, things went well when I moved into his apartment and found a job right away. We began talking about marriage in six months. We had a small wedding; I sent Mom a telegram from our honeymoon in Atlanta, since I knew she wouldn't approve.

Edmond was six feet two, with massive legs, blond hair, blue eyes. A comical guy, except when he was drunk -- then he would pick a fight with anyone. He had the unfortunate combination of being a mean drunk and a terrible fighter. Edmund came home with his face looking like hamburger. When we lived in Memphis, he arrived one night looking particularly mauled. His mother was coming to visit, so I put makeup all over his swollen head and black eyes. Like most of our relationship, it was a futile effort. When his mother walked in our apartment, the first thing she said was, "Who did you get in a fight with?"

When we were together, drinking and partying, the future looked bright. Edmond would bet $5,000 over whether the sun was going to rise in the morning. He loved the excitement and buzz of the gamble. One New Year's Day, he bet that a certain player would score in the third quarter. I said we would split the money if we won. We did, and he gave me half the winnings, which I took and bought a diamond. Of course, his money was gone the next day. But he loved telling the story and that I did something with the winnings. Edmond was proud of his pretty wife, and I knew he loved me.

A year after we were married, we were transferred to the Midwest, to Omaha. He was promoted to district manager and would be traveling five states. My company transferred me to a similar position in Nebraska. Omaha was a drinking man's town, and Edmond fit in well.

On a Friday night, he asked me to pick him up at the airport after a convention in Palm Springs. I got there on time, Edmond's luggage arrived, but he was a no show. Three days later, he called me from Las Vegas and said he was having a ball. He asked me to pick him up in another three days. His baggage didn't even get there this time. Two days later, the call was from Reno. When he eventually found Omaha, I lost my way to the airport and let him think his luggage was lost for a few more days.

It was just weeks later when I saw him on the way home from work. Edmond was crossing the street, holding the arm of our next-door neighbor's wife as they went into a tavern for a drink. Their eyes met mine and we all knew. I was broken and utterly alone, but I had been alone for a while. Edmond was traveling three weeks in a row; most of the time he was days late coming home. He didn't even try to wash away the lipstick and makeup I found on his shirts. I knew he was doing it because of his drinking.

I was a thousand miles from home, married to a man my mother despised, so I made the best of things. I couldn't run home; Mom was the last person I would ever call. She was so opposed to us getting married. She always hated him; they hated each other. I was 29 years old, alone in a strange town and for the first time in my life, second-guessing my decisions.

I stopped taking birth control pills, thinking that if I had a baby, I wouldn't be so alone. I wanted it so badly; I even thought it might change Edmond. When I did get pregnant the following year, Edmond was thrilled, but he kept drinking. Then his anger turned toward me. Strong as an ox, he would grab my hands. Twisting my wrists in a vise lock, he blamed me for who he was.

Tennie was born six weeks early and weighed less than five pounds when we left the hospital. Two months later, she developed salmonella. They never figured out where it came from. My mother visited for the first time and stayed for two weeks. His mom helped for another two.

It was during these days when I first felt what would later be defined as depression. I was sitting in the hospital's nursery, glass walls on every side, wondering, "Was it my fault?" "Was it his fault?" "Whose fault was it?"

When Tennie was six months old, we were transferred to Nashville for a year, then on to Memphis. The sad hopelessness grew worse. When Edmond was out of town, I was afraid to be alone. A friend with three children, whose husband was also out of town, let me stay with her. I was awake during the night, wondering where Debby might have some pills I could overdose on. The feeling was of being overwhelmed, worthless, wanting to just dissolve and disappear. Debby called my husband and together they decided I should be hospitalized. I felt overwhelmed by just living and feeling worthless about myself. I just wanted to disappear. I didn't really want to hurt myself; I just wanted to dissolve. It was terrible.

Debby kept Tennie while I was in the mental hospital. The first night, my roommate set our room on fire and then blamed it on me. The following night, she did the same thing. This time, after the fire department left, Edmond came and took me home. I went back to North Carolina with my mother. Calm only in the midst of chaos, she took control: "I will get you a doctor, a hospital, anything you need." She took me to Charlotte, where I was hospitalized and given electro-shock treatments.

We were transferred back to Nashville, where we bought a two-story house. Edmond didn't have to travel, but nothing else changed. He stayed out late some nights and didn't come home at all on others. I was sure there was at least one girlfriend. Finally, I packed my bags in the night and moved back in with my mother.

Tennie turned 3 in North Carolina. I was prescribed anti-depressants and tranquilizers. In a few weeks, I began to feel better. I flew back to Nashville, sold the house, and brought Edmond to Charlotte, where we rented an apartment together. I quickly found a job as a receptionist, but Edmond grew depressed, unable to find a job. I was working, taking Tennie to day care, buying the groceries and taking care of everything.

A year later, Edmond was still unemployed, spending his days reading, smoking, and watching television; there wasn't enough money for drinking. Then one afternoon, he told me he had an interview in Dallas and would be flying out in the morning. I felt a bit of hope until I called the airport and asked what time his flight number arrived at Dallas. They said it ended in Nashville. And so it did.

When he returned, Edmond confessed he was with a girlfriend in Nashville. I lost it and threw him and his clothes out of the apartment. Edmond left for parts unknown, never paying child support.

The same year, I was visiting my cousin on Thanksgiving afternoon when her husband and a friend came in from the Christmas parade where they had been working as volunteer policemen. I was introduced to the friend, Charlie. He was good looking and the exact opposite of Edmond — small and thin with short, dark hair. My cousin excitedly called the next day and said that Charlie was a lawyer, that he was divorced and would like to ask me out for dinner if I was interested. This began another love in my life. He had a 7-year-old son by his previous marriage who visited every other weekend. Our children got along well. A year and a half later, we married and bought a house near his office.

My father died during this time when he was only 63 -- too many years of drinking and smoking. Mom became very lonely and wanted to visit more often.

Charlie had three meals on the table every day when he wanted them. I was cooking all the time and never knew how many to prepare for as he was always inviting friends without calling ahead. He began to drift into a masculine world I could not enter — the Navy and police Reserves, a gun club, an auto club. He spent endless hours in his garage working on old Corvette. Once, he had 13 of them.

When the depression returned, I immediately went to a local psychiatrist, who prescribed anti-depressants, and I talked with my pastor, who suggested a Christian counselor. I was grasping for all the help I could get, something that was normal for me.

Charlie began drinking vodka and taking two Equagecis at night so he could sleep; my psychiatrist thought this was an unusual habit. Charlie didn't understand my illness or why I had to see a counselor or take a prescription. I had to take care of myself.

Things got better as I struggled to make life normal. Then Tennie began to have anxiety attacks. She was only in the third grade but would stay up late into the night. Despite getting little sleep, she became an over-achiever in school, always bringing home a good report card. Charlie was short-tempered with Tennie; I didn't know what to do. I took her to a school counselor, then a therapist through church; finally, Tennie met with a private child counselor. It seemed helpful for both of us.

Mom met a widower, and they were married a year after my father died. She sold her house and lived on her new husband's farm. They went to London for their honeymoon, and for the first time in my life, I thought my mother was going to be happy.

I loved Charlie, but I could never seem to please him. He was never satisfied with my hairstyle. If it was short, he wanted it long; if it was blonde, he wanted me to be a brunette. I was trying desperately to give him what he wanted, but we grew further apart, never taking a vacation during the ten years we were married.

Toward the end, my sister-in-law called to tell me that my brother had a massive heart attack and that I should come. I spent a week with Jimmy and his family in Alabama. Two weeks after I left, he died; he was only fifty-one.

I was devastated, but Charlie didn't even try to help. I just wanted someone I could hold at night; I needed him to be my best friend, someone I could talk to about Jimmy. He said he couldn't relate and just couldn't feel those things.

It ended when a friend told me that Charlie was sleeping with my first cousin and bragging about it in the family. I simply told him that I wanted a divorce, because I didn't love him anymore. He asked how long I felt this way, and I said it had been several years. I never told him I knew his little secret.

Six months later, Tennie couldn't sleep and was crying again.She became defiant, just doing what she wanted, watching TV, eating, going to the movies whenever she wanted. I took her to a psychiatrist who specialized in adolescents. She was only in eighth grade, but her psychiatrist placed her in hospital for a month.

While Tennie was away, I ran into an old friend at the mall. Walter didn't know I was separated and said he would like to date.

We started going out, and at the end of the one-year waiting period, I went alone to court, secured the uncontested divorce, bought a bottle of champagne, wrapped it in the divorce papers, and delivered it to my ex-husband's office. We are still friends.

The first few years went well for Tennie and me. She adjusted to a new school and made new friends; I was busy with my job, a new house, and dating.

When Tennie was a senior, she was hospitalized again for anxiety and depression. Then, an MRI revealed a brain tumor that required surgery. The tumor was an astrocytoma in the stem of the brain. The neurosurgeon was unable to remove all of it. They recommended 30 radiation treatments. It was a long, painful recovery. Mom helped us tremendously, taking Tennie to her daily radiation treatments.

The worry of all this was more than I could handle. I wanted to be strong, and when Tennie got sick, I tried to stay strong so I wouldn't worry her. Yet, the depression flowed over me again. Tennie and I were both going for counseling and taking antidepressants. It wasn't long before we were both in the same hospital.

Thoughts of suicide came so often I couldn't think of anything else. In one of my better times, I sold the two guns in the house so I wouldn't turn them on myself.

Tennie left for college ninety miles from home, and I was alone for the first time in years. The depression poured over me again. I fought it by getting involved in a singles group at church.

Gardening became a new hobby, and I could feel the calmness of the exercise it gave.

I continued to date Walter; we usually went out for dinner on Friday and Saturday evenings. In a city known for its car dealerships owned by race car drivers and celebrities, Walter owned more dealerships than anyone. And he loved his toys — airplanes, sailboats, and season tickets to all the pro games. We had a great time together.

Then my stepfather had to enter a nursing home and died after a series of health problems. Mom was alone again, and the burden was on me. I became overwhelmed by suicidal thoughts. I just wanted to go to sleep and drift away. I took an overdose of prescription drugs; a friend found me and I was hospitalized again for my own safety.

The same psychiatrist treated me for ten years. During an appointment in November of the tenth year, he said to me, "I have decided depression is the worst illness in the world." I looked into his eyes and realized he was talking about himself. The next month he took his own life.I went to his funeral staggering under the thought, "Here was one of the most successful and admired physicians in the city."

Walter and I had been dating for fifteen years when he sent me a "Dear John" letter saying he had met another lady whom he planned to marry. He hoped I had a nice life.

I felt myself losing my battle with depression. Walter was a powerful man in town, and I was consumed with thoughts that he might try to hurt me to get rid of that part of his life.I took another bottle of pills and was hospitalized once again. My internist recommended that I see Dr. Sethi. With the right combination of medications the anxiety began to lesson and I was no longer washed away by the little things.

At the age of 62, I try to keep a positive attitude in my ongoing battle with depression. My mom is living with me now. She is 88 and in good health. My daughter is 31; she is in the care of a good doctor and doing well.

Psychiatric Assessment

Mollie was clearly suffering from depression when she first came to my office. For several weeks, she said, she had been feeling "very depressed" and had been sleeping poorly — she had trouble falling asleep and woke often during the night. She felt very lethargic, had "no energy" and hadn't eaten well for over a week. She was confused at work and had difficulty with her short-term memory. She hadn't gone to work for two or three days, and wasn't keeping up with her household activities.

Mollie was clearly dysphoric. From the Greek, "dusphoros," dysphoria literally means "hard to bear." It is a state of malaise where depression often triggers anxiety.Her body movements and thinking were slow, showing signs of psychomotor retardation. However, her memory and concentration were intact. She was cooperative and made good eye contact; her speech was linear and goal-oriented. She was alert to place, time, and those around her, and said she was not suffering from paranoia, hallucinations, or delusions, although she mentioned that she felt like people were watching her at work.

Mollie has been afflicted with depression since she was in her 30s. She's aware of the situation, but at her first visit, she said she couldn't remember significant events in her life including specific episodes of her illness. She did recall being hospitalized at least seven times in a psychiatric hospital and most recently placed by her internist in a psychiatric unit of a regional hospital. She had been prescribed Prozac, Elavil, Paxil and Zoloft, and had begun taking St. John's Wort and Lithium Carbonate.

Since her psychiatrist committed suicide, she went to few other psychiatrists, but did not feel comfortable, and thus went back to her Internist. He has been urging her to seek help from a mental health professional.

Because of her poor recall, I was unsure if she met the criteria for Bipolar Affective Disorder. She has a significant family history of depression. Her mother and grandmother suffered depression, and Mollie's daughter, who is in her late twenties, has been hospitalized for depression and is currently being treated with Zoloft. Mollie also has a history of repeated suicide attempts by overdosing on her medications. But on this day, she denied having any suicidal thoughts or intent. She said she wasn't taking drugs or abusing alcohol, didn't smoke or ingest excessive amounts of caffeine. She was taking Premarin as a post-menopausal hormone treatment.

There was a minor oddness in her appearance, which made me suspicious she may be suffering mild psychotic features that may not have been treated by her other psychiatrists. On a scale of one to 10, 10 being the best and I being the worst, she rated her overall functioning around one and her depression at two.

We discussed her personal history: Her childhood was "OK," but she remembers suffering significant physical and emotional abuse from her father and cousin who were both alcoholics. She has been divorced twice, from marriages of ten and eight years. She has one grown daughter and has been in a long-term relationship with a 64-year-old man for the past 13 years. She works for an insurance company. Her current stressors are her daughter moving in with her, the recent recurrence of depression, and an affair she had more than 30 years ago. She cites as her support system her long-term companion and a good job.

My initial diagnosis was that Mollie had a severe and recurrent Major Depressive Disorder. I ruled out Major Depressive Disorder with psychotic features as well as Bipolar Affective Disorder.

I educated her on her psychiatric condition as well as the medications and their potential side effects, recommending she discontinue the St. John's Wort and the Effexor her internist had given her. I prescribed instead Remeron 15 mg before sleep and continued the low dose of Lithium Carbonate 300 mg per day. A follow up appointment was scheduled for three days.

Based on her suicidal history, I would have preferred to recommend hospitalization for her safety and treatment. But since she denied being suicidal, I knew she would no longer fulfill the new "Medical Necessity" criteria required by insurance companies for admission. A Partial Hospitalization during the day would have been appropriate, but there is typically a one to two-week waiting period for admission. Thus the best we could do was to schedule Mollie for frequent office visits.

Follow up Sessions

Mollie's 85-year-old mother, who had accompanied her on her first visit, returned for the second session with the patient. Mollie had only taken the Remeron for one night and was still taking the St. John's Wort along with the Lithium. She said she hadn't had any suicidal thoughts or intentions, but she was extremely anxious, saying her past few days at home were very bad. She stared intensely at me with the same oddness as during her first visit. I told her not to drive, to be with someone all the time, to remove any guns or lethal weapons from her home. I doubled her dose of Remeron and prescribed a low dose of Alprazolam 0.25 mg to take for anxiety. We scheduled another visit for a few days later.

At the third visit, Mollie admitted she had taken her medications only sporadically. She tried going back to work, but felt so anxious she returned home. She was not eating and sleeping only when she took the Remeron, so I tried to educate her again about the chronic nature of her illness, reminding her that it's been with her for years and that she's got to take her medicine if she's going to feel better.

At the fourth session, Mollie had started taking the medications on a regular basis. She said she felt 20% better, but one day she felt hypomanic and impulsively bought clothes from a thrift store. She was unable to drive and function, so I wrote her a medical leave for work. The Lithium Carbonate was increased to 600 mg at night and the Remeron to 45 mg.

Ten days later, Mollie said she was tolerating the increased dosages and was sleeping and eating better. She denied any manic urges to buy excessive and unnecessary items, but she was feeling discouraged because she was not feeling better. I encouraged her to start driving and begin work part time. I explained the role of antipsychotic medications, and began her on a low dose of Risperdal 0.5 mg at night.

In another 10 days, Mollie's mood had improved. She drove herself to the office for the first time, and there was a glimpse of a smile on her face. She was eager to return to work. Her daughter had moved out, and her mother was planning to return to her own home. Overall, Mollie was feeling optimistic and denied any suicidal thoughts.

Two weeks after that visit, Mollie said she had returned to work and was performing at about 80 to 90% of her ability. She was cleaning and cooking at home, and her anxiety, depression, and paranoia at work were improving. Her sleep and appetite were returning to normal levels, and she had gained a few pounds. We were both encouraged by her progress.

A month later, Mollie admitted to feeling a lot of stress at home. She said she stopped watching television because of the "bad news." She was also waking up at night having an "anxiety attack." Mollie reduced the Lithium from 600 mg to 300 mg on her own.Several days before I had also received a phone call from the pharmacy that there might be a negative drug interaction with the Lithium and Risperdal. I told the pharmacist that I would be attentive to any side effects, but was not overly concerned as the dosages were very small. However, Mollie was *very* concerned about a possible interaction. I reassured her that the chances were extremely small and warned that it was far more dangerous for her to adjust her own medication. I recommended that she begin to see a psychotherapist, and we scheduled a follow up visit for 30 days. But she called two weeks later to say that she had quit taking the Lithium and developed a rash. She wanted to discontinue the Risperdal as well. I reluctantly agreed.

At the next visit, Mollie's mood was mildly dysphoric – she was anxious and fearful. She had been seeing a Christian counselor at a local church and was only taking the Remeron and Alprazolam. She was very anxious when alone, and so fearful of the world news that she stopped the newspaper.Her weight had dropped five pounds in the past month. I encouraged her to continue the medications and started a low dose of Haloperidol 0.5 mg at night, and we scheduled an appointment in two weeks.

She didn't show up for that appointment, and I didn't hear anything from her. A copy of her internist's notes arrived at my office two weeks later:

> *Complex 59-year-old female with major psychiatric disturbance as outlined in extensive chart, managed*

recently by Dr. Sethi of psychiatry, presents as urgent work-in today. Complaints of classic somatic manifestations of inadequately controlled Major Depressive Disorder. She had an exhaustive work-up of these symptoms in the past including CBC, thyroid profile, and a metabolic profile that was normal. She had a brain MRI performed by a neurologist, showing only a small thalamic lacunae, consistent with age, modest hyperlipidemia, etc. He felt her memory problems were related to her major depression. She had seen another neurologist two years before. There is no objective reason to look further for hidden organic disease. She describes classic nonspecific light-headedness, lethargy, fatigue, early morning awakening, decreased concentrating ability, forgetfulness, and lost of appetite. These symptoms have been worse in the past two weeks, not coincidently associated with the onset of the holidays. Dr. Sethi discontinued her Lithium though she has been on this for years. She had no adverse metabolic problems with it. She is on the maximum dose of Remeron and estrogen replacement. She is on a fairly low dose of Risperdal, and has had some psychotic thinking in the past. I am hesitant to increase her Xanax. She states she needs refills. She has not scheduled a follow up appointment with Dr. Sethi, and is frustrated she has failed to make major progress with "Christian Counseling."

Tried to emphasize there is no objective or organic explanation for her symptoms. It would be unfair to her to pursue an exhaustive and expensive esoteric work-up in light of this, and strongly recommend she resume seeing Dr. Sethi.

Nine months after I received this note, Mollie came to my office. She had been hospitalized for four days after overdosing on 30 Unisom sleeping pills. After being released, she saw a psychiatrist at the local Mental Health facility emergency room who prescribed Klonopin 1 mg — half in the morning and half at night -- and continued the Remeron 45 mg she was taking. In the intervening months, her internist was prescribing her medications.

Mollie says she overdosed on the Unisom after her companion of 15 years wrote her a note that he was in love with another woman. She was further stressed by her brother-in-law's suicide in January. Additionally, after experiencing numerous medical problems, her 86-year-old mother moved back in with her, and her daughter was getting married in two months.

She was very anxious, staring intensely, and was very guarded. She had gained 18 pounds since her last visit. Once again, I explained the psychiatric illness and its history as well as the critical need for her to continue taking her medications. Mollie was not sleeping, and despite her recent episode, she denied any suicidal thoughts. I restarted her on Risperdal 0.5 mg, and Trazodone 50 mg for sleep as needed. I also consulted with her internist and shared my treatment plan, and explained that due to her long standing psychiatric history, she must be treated by a psychiatrist she feels comfortable with.

At the next session, Mollie was still grieving from the break-up of her 15-year relationship. She had returned to work after being out for three weeks. On reviewing the medications, it was clear Mollie has done well on Lithium and Alprazolam, thus these were started again.

In subsequent sessions, Mollie has made steady progress. Due to her weight gain, the Remeron was substituted with Effexor with a good response. She started Christian counseling again and was able to withstand multiple stressors without a relapse. Her work at the insurance company is going well, and Mollie is now able to drive five hours to see her daughter at her new home. I substituted her Lithium with Topamax, and she is losing weight. Currently, Mollie is stable on Effexor XR 75 mg, Risperdal 0.5 mg, Topamax 100 mg, and Trazodone 50 mg. She is functioning well, and she is scheduling visits every six to eight weeks.

The ancient Romans had a saying that sometimes it is heroic merely to endure. There are heroes among us. People like Mollie who daily fight an illness that is little understood by those around them and even by themselves, and by people who feel a shame that society still places a stigma on mental illness. In this environment, they are led to believe that they would not need medications if only they were strong enough or trying hard enough. They believe they should be able to fight it on their own. We would be ashamed to place such burdens on a person suffering from cancer, heart disease or AIDS. Yet, the ancient fears and stigmas remain. It is time we see these people as heroes, individuals who are doing incredible feats each morning as they arise and bravely face a new world.

CHAPTER 7

How Sad and Bad and Mad It Was

We loved, sir—used to meet:
How sad and bad and mad it was—
But then, how it was sweet!

Robert Browning

I am tired of being sad; I had a beautiful giggle, now my heart is split in two. It will take time to heal. I am clean now, I don't want to be dirty; it's like being gay. I drove tanks at Ft. Knox and loved the discipline of the Army. I loved being clean, perfect, with my brass shined; I shined all my bars until they glowed.

I want to travel, go to Niagara Falls, then to California and see the Sequoia trees; I can't wait to see them. I want a house in St. Martins or Bermuda where I can go two or three times a year. I have already bought a Ford Ranger pickup, all new clothes, new shirts. I am tired of being sad.

My name is Lee. My life seemed to begin when I was 6 years old in Freemont, Ohio. While my parents slept, I climbed down the silver metal bars of the TV antenna, off and running as soon as I hit the ground. At first, we darted through mom-and-pop corner stores, stealing a bottle of cheap wine — Mad Dog 20/20 or Thunderbird. Then we began lifting cases of beer.

We would roam the streets, making it back before morning. Climbing my TV ladder, crashing before Mom woke us up for school. My days in elementary school were spent sleeping in class, then smarting off at my teachers and causing trouble when I was awake. After a while, both sides gave up. I would just walk to the office, where I would pick up my detention slip or hear the call to my parents telling them I was expelled. At home, Mom and Dad would see who could hit me the hardest, throw me the farthest. But it helped me in the street; I knew how to take a beating.

Because of all this, my brother decided he would have a piece of me. David is only one year older but has always been twice my size. It was the same each night. I went to bed at 9:00, and then he would come in and wait, lying in his bed — waiting behind me. When the house was quiet, he would come, lie on top of me and rape me while his hand held my mouth. It seemed like 15 minutes; it could have been longer, maybe a few moments. I cried; I hurt; I bled. It ended with, "I'll kill you if you say anything to anyone, and I'll tell Mom and Dad you have been doing this to me." It was the same night, every night, for two years

During the day, David threatening to kill me if I talked, I shined his shoes and washed the dishes he was supposed to do. He is still six inches taller, divorced for the fourth time; his liver is gone.

My sister Mary is two years younger. She is very tiny. I protected her for 15 years while I was home. My dad was a little fat truck driver — always wired, any little sound could fire him up. He would throw food off the table. I would hide and run, but he beat my mother. Mary and I would hide. I resent Mother for staying with Dad; he punched me in the mouth. I had nightmares of grabbing my sister by her hair, and I would be my momma and she would lie in my arms. Mary left home only to marry another man who beat her. She was abused for so long she doesn't even have a self to have confidence in. She is just there, married to an alcoholic, just there.

The only way out was through drugs — a moment of peace away from time and pain. My first love was pot, then acid; I fell for any drug that was on the market. I was so far behind in my education; I thought I was ahead. The pain became real again after one too many run-ins with the law. Friends pealed away as I became too dangerous to hang with.

I decided to leave home at 15, and rented my first house trailer for 65 bucks a month. I still went to school when I wasn't working, but I started drinking at work and after school — drugging out the rest of the night. Those who say you have to hit bottom before you can get better don't know that it can always get worse. Too many troubles. They "asked" me to leave school six months before graduation.

At 17, there were no options until a recruiter said I could be a mechanic in the Army. The first year went well. I learned about tanks, weapons, and enjoyed the discipline. It even felt good to be told what to do and when. Fort Knox was a good place. Then off to Fort Sill for advanced training — bigger tanks, guns, more discipline. It was a good life until I found the druggies and the drunks. My best friend was on guard duty when he ripped off a stereo from one of the best soldiers in the company. After they arrested Ted, the MPs took me into a bare room with a cement floor and steel table. They locked the door and told me to strip. I passed out after the second MP raped me. I was alone when I woke, pulling on my pants as the blood dripped out of me.

I went to the base doctor who told me I was just a little red and told me to return to my unit. Once again, there was no one to tell, no family to call. There was only one choice — to overdose. I decided to have a goodbye party with enough drugs for everyone and too many for me. This was my way out. I even screwed this up; no one was interested in anything I had to offer. This was not how it was supposed to be. I began taking all the pills myself until the people at the party became concerned and dropped me in front of the Commander's guardhouse. Somehow I managed to walk away from the guardhouse that night until I passed out in the marching field. The base chaplain found me alongside the path on his morning run.

It was only for a moment, but someplace in that clouded field I found it, the peace that I had never felt; it was just for a second, too brief to hold on to. I woke up three days later in the intensive care unit. Arthur, the chaplain, hung around after I left the hospital, wondering why I was so sure I wanted to die at 18 years old. As we talked about my family and spoke of Dad, he asked why I wrote that my father was dead on my enlistment papers. Arthur really seemed to care, but there was too much guilt to tell the whole story. Guilt about letting my father hurt Mom, guilt for being raped, and then now, the other feelings.

A few months later I was firing Howitzers in Vietnam. I came back to the States as we all did — feeling the bewildering disgrace of having been to that place. The best thing I could do is not tell anyone about my Army days; again, it was something I kept in the closet.

I returned to the same gas station I left when I was 15. I met a girl named Karen. It was wonderful — all-night parties, nightclubs until they threw us out, shared hangovers as we stumbled around the next day. We had seven wonderful wild years of fun: drinking, hell raising, and doing drugs. We bought our first house and discovered all our neighbors were into the same lifestyle; it was magnificent.

The party ended when Karen's father decided to open a supermarket in another town with the promise that he would hire everyone in the family. Karen already decided before I was ever told. I was betrayed.

But looking for our new house was fun. As neighbors came to say hello, I started feeling this was a good thing. We worked through long nights to open the store. Then, a day before the grand opening, Karen's dad said he thought it might become a problem for the in-laws to work in the store; it would be only family. Once again, it was an act of betrayal.

A few weeks went by until I got the courage to look for a job. I was hired to pump gas; the worst part was that my wife was making more money than me.We never talked about it because I knew she was working hard to make the store a success. And I began to make friends and became so good at selling extra stuff at the pumps that my boss made me a manager. I was making 10 percent of my sales, and this finally brought me close to what Karen was making. I found the local drug dealers, discovering my boss was the main cocaine dealer in town. I was only smoking pot at the time, which was fine as he was able to keep me in stock. Life seemed to be good. Until Karen came home with a look I had never seen on her face. She had just had a long talk with her Dad; they decided it was time for us to start a family.

I felt controlled; even worse, with her parents' support Karen said the booze and drugs had to stop. I stayed straight while we were trying to conceive. When Karen became pregnant, we were excited about everything: Getting the baby room ready, filling the dresser with little clothes, hanging toys around the crib, talking in bed at night about what we would name our child.

Things were good. A new job with a national sales company was going better than I could have dreamed. I was driving a company car and finally making more money than my wife. What a life!

The joy of driving to the hospital while Karen was in labor overcame any fears and doubts. But then it was night. Some force of evil, and the doctor's forceps, crushed our son as he entered the world. It was briefly explained that his skull might not have been fully developed.

The pain was so deep we couldn't look at each other. Karen's family needed something to blame, so they chose me. I was the one who took drugs and was a drunk. "You killed your own child."

I took every pill and drank every bottle of liquor I could find and drove alone until I didn't know where I was. Maybe it was my fault. Maybe I'm not fit to be a parent or a decent husband.

Like the night on the Army parade ground, by some weird bend of grace, I found myself sitting in a tent revival. Ron was a missionary who happened to be there. He sat next to me, looked me in the eyes, and said "Go home." Whatever he meant, I took it as a command. For a moment, once again clarity came uninvited and unexpected. I talked with Karen for the first time in days, and I was able to lay down the things that were said about me.

We decided we would try again; this time it was our decision. Years passed, our sons Tommy and Will are getting older now, staying overnight with friends. When they were still young, I was driving a truck for a living. Coming home one night, a crash shot me through the window into the highway median. The following months were filled with operations and hospitals. Remarkably, it also opened a whole new world of drugs. I could have any kind, any time, all I had to do was ask. It was easy to play doctors off against each other. I worked up to Oxycontin. I didn't know it was known as "red-neck heroin" until my chiropractor told me kids were crushing it and snorting it.

Great news for a drug addict. As soon as I got home, I was sitting on the toilet cutting up my pills with a razor blade. Karen walked in. The guilt, pain, blaming, and avoidance crushed me. I was committed to the psychiatric unit of our local hospital.

A few days later, my doctor called and said my blood tested positive for Hepatitis C. It broke Karen; we couldn't even mention it. She moved into another bedroom, stopped making dinner and washing my clothes. She would not even sit next to me. I began taking interferon shots every Friday, and the medication made me so sick all I could do was sleep through the weekends.

My mind began to unravel. The only thing I could focus on was killing myself. If I tried to concentrate, thoughts would bind me to the sadness of childhood.I was finally under a psychiatrist's care. I began to tell him the things that had haunted me for years — my desires to be . . . I still refuse to bear the thought of being gay or bisexual. I just want to be a mother, take care of others, or give a hug to a person with cancer. It felt right. Being gay is not me, being a woman would make the thoughts and desires normal.

I begged Karen to come with me to the psychiatrist so she could have some idea of what was happening to me. All she would say is that I was the one who was sick, not her. I started a water treatment business, mainly digging and repairing septic tanks; it was going well. But I was so sick from the hepatitis that I had to force myself to get up just to keep the business going. I lost seventy pounds and told Karen that I couldn't do this on my own, but she turned away.

In June 2003, I filed for divorce and moved a trailer onto some property we owned next to our house. My pastor visited me a few months later and said I would have to give up my volunteer work in the church. I had been teaching an adult class and leading the Promise Keepers group. Karen and her friend were spreading rumors that I had a bomb and planned to blow up the church.

There was also talk that I was wearing woman's clothes. My pastor said he didn't have a choice.

There was just too much: the divorce, hepatitis, my company, worrying if my sons loathed me, and my own self-hatred. When I got angry I would say, "Poor me, you are not worthy of God, of forgiveness and mercy." At its worst, the depression brought me to a place where I began to starve myself, thinking "This is a way out without hurting anyone." It would seem as if I died of natural causes. I lost 70 pounds in six weeks.I began shaking uncontrollably.

Even though I did not feel worthy enough to be breathing — even here — there were friends, people who stepped between death and me. They set a net around me, making sure there was someone with me every day and in the evenings. They made suppers and stayed until I ate. But even friends could not stop my mind from crumbling.

Moments became increasingly disconnected. The rooms in my trailer no longer made sense or had a purpose. I would walk into the bathroom with no idea why I was there. But once again, when there was nothing left, God sent a friend.A man from my former church began to come by every evening. When we spoke, it was just small talk, most of the time he just sat with me. One night he said, "I think you are doing better." His very words began to heal. "Yes, I am getting better. I can do some things without constant thoughts of taking my life."

There is always hope. It helps if you are near those who are hopeful, those who believe that no person is beyond God's mercy.

The small things keep me connected to friends and life. Making sure the house is clean, staying straight, going to AA meetings, and sitting with a friend.

The good thing is I am tired of being sad. But of course, it will take time to heal.

Psychiatric Assessment and Follow Up

When Lee came to my office, he was 47 years old, 5-foot-8, very slender. He weighed 162 pounds, dressed in very brief shorts and a tight fitting T-shirt. He was clean-shaven, tanned, and his short dark hair was slicked back in odd-looking patches. He was referred by a friend who is a therapist, and he was clearly anxious.

He was severely nervous, waking up early and unable to return to sleep. He had a lack of sexual desire, difficulty attaining an erection. He has been married for 25 years and has two teenage sons. His wife Karen manages their business. They have been having marital problems and Lee believes they will separate. They have not had sex in more than six months.

Lee told a painful story of trauma and substance abuse. His father emotionally and physically abused him. He has had no contact with his parents for 15 years. He has a younger sister. An older brother raped him when Lee was eight. His brother also has a lifetime history of substance abuse.

Lee quit school when he was a junior and joined the Army at 17.After six military police raped him, leaving him unconscious, and bleeding from his rectum and mouth, he tried to commit suicide by overdosing on pills. After an examination, the military physician reported that he was not raped. Following his suicide attempt, he was hospitalized in a psychiatric ward for three weeks.

There is a history of severe substance abuse. Lee began drinking when he was 8, with his heaviest drinking from the ages of 17 to 30. He abused numerous drugs including cocaine, LSD, intravenous heroin, marijuana, opiods, and cigarettes. It is likely this abuse is related to the symptoms of Post Traumatic Stress Disorder originating from his sexual, physical, and emotional trauma. Lee has been sober for more than six years and attends AA and NA meetings on a regular basis.

He was diagnosed with fibromyalgia a year ago. Six months later his physician told him he was suffering from Hepatitis C. He was treated with Zenaflex, Prednisone, Skelexin, Oxycontin, and Percocet. He stopped these medications and continues to take Ribavarin and Interferon for the Hepatitis. In addition, he takes Zantac and Prevacid for gastric ulcers, and Tylenol as needed for pain.

He was recently hospitalized when he became severely depressed and suicidal. He has been under the care of a psychiatrist who treated him with Celexa and Remeron.

I gave a diagnosis of Major Depressive Disorder, marital stress, and a history of Polysubstance Dependence.I continued his current medications and strongly recommended he keep seeing his therapist; we scheduled a second session in two weeks.

At this session, Lee's depression and anxiety were more severe as his marriage was deteriorating. He wanted to see a different therapist than his neighbor who was currently treating him.

I increased the Remeron to 45 mg, and prescribed a low dose of Alprazolam as needed for anxiety. I gave him a recommended list of therapists and stressed that he must continue therapy.

After this visit, I received a call from Lee's oncologist, who wanted to make sure that Lee continued to see me because one serious side effect of the Interferon is severe depression as well as suicidal thoughts. Many patients receiving this medication, without also receiving antidepressants, have indeed committed suicide. With permission, I shared Lee's complicated psychosocial stressors with his oncologist to ensure Lee received the best-informed medical care.

At his third visit, three weeks later, Lee's was doing better. He was seeing a new therapist, his business was doing well, and he was considering reconciliation with his wife. However, this stage in his recovery was brief. When Lee came the following month he recounted many problems: suffering from diarrhea and back pain, was irritable and depressed, and was having problems with the phone at work. At this session, he recounted an issue that obviously brought him severe stress. Lee was quite confused with his sexual identity. Unsure if he was gay or bisexual, he practiced cross-dressing: He enjoyed shaving his legs, wearing pantyhose and women's clothing. His therapist encouraged him to discuss this issue with me. Lee was specific in relating that he was not happy in his own body as a man. He denied being suicidal. I increased his Remeron to 60 mg, and recommended him to a therapist who specialized in sexual issues.

At the next visit Lee was facing increasingly difficult psychosocial stressors. Conflicts with his wife escalated until she called the police and charged him with domestic violence. He spent a night in jail and said it was the most humiliating experience of his life. Despite these traumas, Lee's mood was better and he appeared to be dealing well with the stress. He added another employee at work, and his business was profitable. He was very anxious of the upcoming court date. I substituted Xanax with Klonopin, which has a longer half-life in the body and thus has an increased lasting affect on anxiety.

Lee was legally separated in the fall. Despite his good mood, he continued to lose weight and had diarrhea. I substituted Celexa with Prozac as it is less likely to irritate the gastrointestinal system.By November, Lee was suicidal and was physically very ill. His weight dropped to 141 pounds. I strongly recommended he admit himself to the hospital, which he did not wish to do, fearing his wife would use it against him in court, which was to hear his case within the week.

A few days later, I saw Lee on an emergency basis. He was not eating, feeling suicidal, and had considered plans to kill himself. I immediately called the hospital and gave the necessary clinical history Lee needed for admission. The admitting nurse informed me that only two psychiatrists were currently admitting patients to the adult unit. All other psychiatrists in private practice had stopped admitting patients to this private hospital because of low reimbursements as well as daily fights with the insurance companies.

I then called the county mental health center and relayed Lee's clinical history. I gave him directions and the telephone number to the hospital and reminded him of his "No Harm" contract. I gave him samples of Celexa, as it had been more effective than the Prozac he was currently taking. Lee went to the hospital, waited 10 hours in the Emergency Room, and was not admitted. No one called me to relate his status or say he had gone home alone.

Lee's experience is typical of our health care system where patients are increasingly being dislocated from those who care for them. It used to be common courtesy for the attending physician to call the referring doctor to receive more background information, update the treatment plan, or send a discharge summary. As insurance companies literally make, or at least force, clinical decisions, there is a growing environment of anger and frustration. Physicians feel helpless as their clinical judgments and decision are not only questioned but also ignored. Nurses and health care professionals often spend the majority of their time staring at computer screens and calling insurance companies rather than caring for the immediate needs of their patients. And of course patients suffer the most as they are denied recommended treatments while they are being shuttled between physicians with progressively less background on their conditions.

Lee came into my office three weeks later. His primary care physician had given him his medications in the meantime. He recently started therapy with a church counselor, and his Interferon and Ribitron treatment for hepatitis C were completed. He enjoyed Thanksgiving with a friend, and his son had come for a visit. With his business continuing to grow, Lee was looking forward to the holidays. My own concerns about his suicidal thoughts were lessened as he progressed.

A month later, Lee was continuing to see the therapist from his church. He was working on his gender identity issues, began attending AA meetings again and reconnected with a sponsor. His next court date was in a few days; he denied any history of violence or that he was a threat to his wife or anyone else. I complied with his request asking me for a letter to the court stating that he did not intend to kill or hurt his wife.

At his next session, Lee said he was experiencing mood swings and all night crying episodes. He was taking Celexa 40 mg, Remeron 30 mg, and iron for anemia. Lee did not want to increase the Remeron to address the mood swings and crying, so I added a low dose of Wellbutrin 100 mg per day. He denied being suicidal as well as making any threats to his wife. Lee's relationship to his children was improving.

His sexual therapy was going well. He was able to masturbate. He liked women's clothing, and had been purchasing panties, sweaters, and bras.

Two days later, I received a call from his therapist saying that Lee was hyper and hypo-manic. I saw him on the same day.

He was highly irritable, short tempered, angry, nervous, and slightly confused. He denied any violent thoughts toward Karen. In light of these symptoms, I started Lee on Depakote in addition to the other medications.

His mood stabilized within two weeks. He was attending NA meetings and started to help three crack addicts. He continued to make progress in therapy; feeling more comfortable with his sexuality and being alone at home. He started to gain weight. He was tolerating the Depakote 500 mg well along with his other medications: Wellbutrin 100 mg twice daily, Remeron 30 mg., and Celexa 20 mg.

In May, Lee had a complete physical examination. His lab tests showed normal liver enzymes. He was continuing his therapy and had no side effects from the medication. He complained of ongoing pain related to rheumatoid arthritis and osteoporosis. In response, I changed his Celexa to Effexor. As he was making satisfactory progress, we scheduled a monthly appointment. His mood is stable as he is taking Remeron 30 mg, Depakote 250 mg, Effexor 150 mg, and Wellbutrin 200 mg.

At his August visit, Lee spoke about telling his story during an AA meeting, and at his church. He feels very proud of his accomplishments in business and his relationship with his sons, who are working with him.

Lee has wanted to be a girl all his life. He received laser treatment to remove hair from his face, arms, and legs. He is wearing pantyhose, bras and make up. He also has found a jeweler who has made him rings and a necklace.He is planning to take estrogen and has located a surgeon who specializes in removing male sexual organs and reconstructing them to resemble female organs. Lee says he has not had sexual relations with anyone for three years and denies being homosexual. While this may appear rather contradictory, becoming a woman for Lee allows him to feel feminine, have relationships with men, and not consider himself homosexual.

As a psychiatrist, I feel it is my duty to stabilize a patient's brain chemistry to normal levels, allowing them to focus on the major issues in their lives: marriage, relationships, religion, economic issues, and yes, even sex changes.

CHAPTER 8

I Thought Life Was Getting Better

I was finally getting a better grip on my life. My abusive husband was in jail. My children were doing well in school, and I was getting good reviews at my job. I had six people working for me. I was paying all my bills and even saving some money. Then I started to deteriorate, gradually but definitely. I didn't know what was wrong. I started to slip in my job. I was not sleeping well; I felt tired and not together mentally. I felt foggy and heavy in my mind. I was not as sharp as I used to be. My supervisor noticed the difference. One day she called me and asked, "What's wrong, Candy?"

I didn't know. I thought life was getting better.

I started crying. I had never cried in front of anyone before. I was ashamed and felt sorry for myself. I had cried and sobbed before and wished God would take me away. But not like this. Now I could cry at the drop of a hat, and could not stop. I was losing my confidence. I could not afford to lose my job. I had to support my three children, and they are good kids. I knew I would do anything to protect them. I would not allow them to be abused or taken away.

My supervisor urged me to see my family doctor. He checked me out, and looked carefully into all the openings in my body -- mouth, nose, ears, eyes, and even my vagina and anus -- to find the cause of my problems. He found nothing, and my blood work, including a urine drug screen, were also negative. He suspected HIV infection, and asked me all sorts of questions regarding my sex life. Did I start my sexual activity at a young age? How many sexual partners have I had? Do I use condoms? Have I ever used street drugs? Have I used needles? Did I have STDs? Was I involved in homosexual activity? Had I had anal sex? Were my sexual partners drug abusers? Did they have any deviance in their sexual practices?

I answered yes to most of them.

My doctor urged me to get an HIV test - just to rule it out. I was determined to resist. They say it is confidential, but it's not. The insurance companies know right away, since they have to pay for it. I know from my job with the healthcare company that many clients' lives have been ruined by that test. I was not going to do it. He gave me some medications for depression. I had side effects of nausea, vomiting, nervousness, and panic attacks. I lost weight. I had to go to the Emergency Room once just to make sure I was not having a heart attack.

My situation did not improve. I was asked to take medical leave and see a psychiatrist. I said, "No way. I am not psycho or loony. My head is all right. I am not hearing voices or seeing things. Why should I go and see a psychiatrist? Only mentally weak people see a shrink. I am strong mentally, and there is nothing wrong with my head."

At the urging of my insurance company, I finally agreed to see a therapist. She was empathetic and listened to my life story. She told me to go to the local psychiatric hospital and get an assessment. I was petrified.

I started praying harder and going to church every day. I started taking more vitamins and tried to become a vegetarian. I went to Bible classes at the church. Nothing was working. The harder I tried, the worse I became. My mind was not working properly. I had difficulty in getting up now. I was sleeping all day and doing nothing except preparing meals for my children. I was starting to have suicidal thoughts; I made plans of how to kill myself. I could use my husband's gun, take an overdose of pills, or just drive over the edge of the road or into the median. I felt scared: No, I can't take my life. I have children, and I have fought to keep them.

I went with my aunt (whom I call my mother because she raised me) to the hospital for the assessment. There were no problems from my insurance company. In fact, they encouraged me to seek help. I was immediately admitted to the inpatient program and assigned a psychiatrist. I was in a daze.

Many staff members came and talked to me. Finally my psychiatrist came and talked to me for over an hour. He asked lots of questions about my symptoms, how and when they began, my childhood history, details about my mother, any sexual, physical, emotional and drug abuses I may have suffered. He also asked me about my marriages, husbands, education, jobs, children, and stresses. I don't remember what I told him, but he made lot of notes and assured me that I would get well. He gave my illness a name, explained it to me and told me about the medicines he was going to give me to treat it. I felt optimistic.

I started to sleep better but remained in my room. The staff urged me to go to group sessions and participate in therapy. I was frightened and did not want anyone to know my inner secrets and pains. Further, I was in no position to listen to other patients' problems. I was physically weak. I had lost 20 pounds in the past two months. I weighed 110 pounds. My skin was pale, and at age 30, I was getting wrinkles. I looked awful. My sex drive was nil. My breasts were sagging. My legs were weak, with no energy. I was worried no man would have me.

After a couple of days, I was no longer suicidal and had started to eat a little. I was resting better at night despite all the turmoil on the units with patients who were alcoholics, drug addicts, hearing voices and having visual hallucinations. Some of the older patients were having problems with memory, and they wandered into other patients' rooms, especially at night. The rooms were not locked, and one night an old fat man without any clothes came into my room wanting sex. I was horrified and yelled for help. Within a few minutes, a staff member came and took him away.

I had terrible nightmares and ugly dreams of my childhood.

The next morning I told my psychiatrist what had happened. He listened patiently and then informed me that my insurance company was not going to give me any more days in the hospital, as I was no longer feeling suicidal. They did not care that I had no help at home, that I had three children to take care of and limited support. I had hardly dealt with any of the issues that had brought me here. I had worked for this company for eight years and saved lots of money for them. They did not care. If I wanted to stay, I had to pay from my pocket $1,200 per day. I called my supervisor, and she called her boss on my behalf pleading for a few more days in the hospital. As a favor, I got a few days of half a day of partial hospitalization, three to four hours a day.

At home, things were rough. My aunt could not handle the children, although they were happy to have me back. I slept well on the medications, and my appetite was coming back. That gave me some strength.

A van from the hospital came to pick me up in the morning, and I met with my psychiatrist every day. He monitored side effects and adjusted my medications. He encouraged me to share childhood and other abuses. As I gathered some physical and mental strength, I told him the following story:

My mother was from Vietnam. I don't know my father. He was a white American. My mother had three other children from different fathers. She was a prostitute. Her parents were from a good family, but because of war she needed a job. She was 15 years old when she went to work in a bar. I was taken away at age 3 to live with my aunt in Hawaii.

My mother moved there later and continued her profession. Lots of men used to come to be with her. Sometimes, there were drug abusers and alcoholics who beat her and wouldn't pay. My mother used to drink and smoke a lot. Normally the children would go to our aunt's place when Mother was busy.

One day I remember a big, wild man wanted oral sex with me. He chased me all around the house and forced me into it. I was horrified and told my aunt. Within a few days I was taken into a convent.

On my 11th birthday my grandfather came as usual to take me out. He bought me lots of clothes, toys and candy. He touched my private parts and asked me to play with his penis. I liked it. He told me this was our secret. I did not tell anyone. He used to pick me up on weekends and take me to isolated places where I would have oral sex with him.

I wanted to be a woman and wear lots of sexy clothes and perfumes. I became rebellious and started to flirt with men. The convent could not handle me, and they let me go to my aunt's place. I had my first sexual intercourse with my cousin, who was four years older than me. It continued for a few years, and then I started going out with other boys in high school. I was called the "Smart Slut" because I was a good student.

After high school, I came to North Carolina with my aunt. I got a job as a sales clerk in a clothing store and started going to the community college. I was still promiscuous until I met my first husband. Gary was 22 and I was 20 when we got married. He was a good provider and had a good job. We had our first daughter, Kris, within a year.

Gary and I used to drink together and smoke pot. He started to drink heavily and was coming home late. One night, he brought his buddy from work. They were drunk, and they both wanted sex. They tied me up and raped me. That was the end of my marriage. I left home with my daughter, and came to my aunt's place.

I went back to school, took courses in medical claims, and was hired by a healthcare system. I worked very hard and soon became a supervisor. But my life was empty, and I started going to bars. I met my second husband, Mike, in a bar. He was good looking and had a good job. We dated for six months and got married within a year. Soon I became pregnant. I had two healthy twin boys, John and Mike Jr.

Things were going well at home and at my job. I felt happy. Mike and I continue to smoke marijuana and drink beer. Sometimes, Mike would bring cocaine home, and he brought home girls from the bar to have sex. He also brought X-rated videos. He wanted me to participate in group sex. Initially I resisted, but I gave in because I liked it, too.

On week-ends, I used to take the kids to my mom's place and have orgies with Mike's friends at home. One day I got a call from Kris's third-grade teacher for an urgent conference. I was shocked to learn that Mike had been sexually abusing Kris for over a year. DSS and the local police got involved. Mike was convicted and sent to jail. We were recommended for therapy. That was about six months ago, when I started going downhill.

My psychiatrist listened to all this very carefully, and told me that it was very important to deal with these issues in therapy, and at AA / NA meetings, where he said I should look for a female sponsor. I followed his recommendations. My therapy is helping me to understand my childhood abuse, depression and addictive behavior. I am trying very hard to be a new person, to be a good mother to my children. I am regaining my emotional and physical strength. I am back at my job full-time. I must succeed. I must be careful for my children's sake. I can't afford to lose. I pray more often for guidance. I am getting better. I have confidence in my doctors.

CHAPTER 9

I Began Asking Myself ..

By

Walter Fore

BEFORE TREATMENT

"As ashamed of myself as I am … a prisoner in my own life – this is the life I created for myself. The choices that I've made have brought me to this point in time. And where I am right now is Hell. I have no control of my future, my life, my career, my love, and my very existence. Where am I supposed to be? What do you want me to do? Who am I? or better yet, Who have I become? What fate do I deserve, what punishment is enough that I won't have to feel this way anymore? Is it where I sleep? Would things be different if I were somewhere else, somebody else? Will the past still keep coming back? No, I haven't forgotten the past, but I am still doomed to repeat it, or even worse -- make bigger mistakes. Why do I still choose to make mistake after mistake? Today I realized again that inside I feel empty, alone, soulless, and hopeless. Can I take control of my future? Can I change my fate?

"With all these thoughts going through my head, over and over again, at some point I started feeling very weak in mind and body. I noticed that when I looked in the mirror I saw a skinny, weak person. Eventually, I realized that my self-image was what I remember myself looking like in my first year of high school. This was compounded by

the hopelessness and fear that was completely taking over my life. This feeling of smallness and weakness is horrifying. I feel helpless, and in my mind's eye I see a weak, afraid, skinny person shaking with fear because I am unable to accept the choices that I had to make to survive and take care of my family. I am becoming very afraid of not knowing what each new minute could bring. And to me, each new minute could be my last. I have lost control of my future, and I don't like what that means. These feelings have become very overwhelming and over powering -- so I start to discuss possible scenarios with myself. You know the voice in your head that you have discussions with. I would plan and play out hundreds of scenarios in my mind throughout the day until I couldn't remember if I had said things aloud or just thought them. I couldn't remember. I have spent day after day pacing these floors in my house discussing –out loud – what I would do, how I would act, and what I would say. Rehearsing these events over and over. I am having trouble determining if it's happened, going to happen, or did I just play out another situation in my mind? I am beginning to believe myself, but to let my guard down would be foolish. If I'm not on top on my 'game' – that is when I'll be most likely cornered. So, am I weak and afraid, or am I strong and prepared? I can't tell at this point, I'm living my life minute by minute – but still, I only see a skinny weak man.

"I have determined that any form of happiness in my life would render me even more vulnerable to the fate that I believe is waiting for me. Any act of intimacy with my wife is out of the question because I don't feel that I deserve that privilege anymore, and it also mean letting my guard down. So I would smile no more, and laugh

no longer. I do not have the ability to appreciate a clear blue sunny day as I feel others do. It really no longer mattered to me about any of those things because to enjoy and appreciate the simple things in life would mean that my defense is down and they will hit me at my weakest point. I know this to be true.

"I have also begun to ask myself, what are all these people so excited about, why do they seem so happy? Eventually, I began to feel sick inside watching everyone drive by in their new cars, going to their new homes and talking on their latest and greatest cell phones. And again, I ask the question, what is so great? If they knew what I knew, and had been through what I've been through – they wouldn't be so happy anymore, would they? More and more I started to close in and shut out the world …I wanted nothing more to do with society, on a personal level or as a whole. It was becoming increasing clear to me that everyone I had ever met was out to get me in some way – (whether for) money, stability, or to lie and cheat me, they all wanted something. And of course, the very real possibility that they were out to harm my family, even worse, murder all of us.

"I know that they have been watching me, listening in on my phone calls and following me everywhere I go. I see people on the street, blocks away, looking at me and talking on their cell phones, and suddenly they hop in a car and leave. People would follow me to my car in public places, always one man first on the left seemingly walking in the direction that I was planning on walking and then another man blindsiding me from the right. I'm aware of what they're trying to do to me. The man on the left was the distraction, while the

man on the right was there to apprehend me while my focus was not on him. These people, on the street corners, following me, sitting in the parking decks, watching me leave from work are very real. I actually ran from them a couple of times. I took elevators to the wrong floor on purpose, ran up the stairs to where my car was parked, all in an effort to try and trick these people.

"At this point, I am becoming aware of the people in the cars behind me, beside me, in front of me. Even the people at the intersections are watching me. ... I believe that these are a network of people tracking my every move and pin-pointing the exact location as to where to corner me. With this mindset, I barricaded myself in my house. I felt safe there, but ... I felt it was a false sense of security -- my house was not impenetrable. I bought security cameras and put a dead-bolt lock on all the doors of my house. A handgun I keep close by, with two large dogs (to) alarm me if someone was approaching my house or trying to get in. The front lawn of the house was off limits between the hours of 3 p.m. until dusk. ... I knew people had to work, so at the earliest they would get off by 3 p.m. and could possibly be waiting for me to come out the front door... However, my back lawn is fenced in, so it's OK for me to be out there with the exception of the corner, where the entry gate is located. Within (this) time frame I constantly look out the windows to make sure no one is outside. It is almost like living two days in one. The first day began at 4a.m., when I would awake from a nightmare about someone trying to kill me or break into my house and harm me. This has been going on for eight months now. This 'first day' would last from 4 a.m. until around 2 p.m. -- always in my mind I'm worrying about the 3 p.m. 'window.' I am not

safe here, I am a 'sitting duck' -- --- in my car, in my house – it's just a matter of time until they come. This 'second day' starts around 3 p.m. until midnight of the next morning, when I finally would drink myself to sleep, in a desperate attempt not to have those dreams again. And of course, 4 a.m. would come and it started all over again.

"I have been considering getting some kind of professional help. But wouldn't that mean letting my guard down or giving myself a false sense of 'everything is OK'? Let alone the fact I would have to come out of my house, get into my car and go somewhere that I don't feel safe. I can't do it – and I'm watching the quality of my life deteriorate in front of me and I am helpless to do anything about it. My family and my wife's family are starting to notice something is not right. And how can I hide this from them? I've given every excuse in the book as to why I can't come over or participate in any function. I think to myself, 'Please don't come over to my house,' and I stop taking any phone calls from anyone.

"My wife comes to me after one of my weekly 'melt downs' and says, 'I have made an appointment to see a doctor.'

"This would be the beginning of understanding a life-long problem that lay just under the surface until a traumatic event 11 months ago drove me to the life I just spoke of.

"I agreed to keep the appointment and began to carefully calculate how I was going to make it to his office with the least amount of exposure to anyone. This was a huge task to undertake, as I would have to drive a very heavily traveled road. I came to the conclusion that it had to be done and it's time to begin facing what I felt was

going to be a difficult road to recovery. I guess what really bothered me was, what if someone saw me go into the office and waited for me to come back out? A sitting duck. This feeling is very real to me and very hard to overcome. It took a preparation of two hours to talk myself into going to his office. Pacing the floors of my house, talking to myself, answering myself, it had all come to this, I could chose to go or chose to stay home where I'm safe and keep living like this.

These feelings are real; this fear is real to me."

Treatment

Paul was referred by his wife, Ann, who had been my patient for over a year. Paul came to my office at the end of August 2003. He was extremely nervous and depressed, and he wanted to stand for a few minutes before he settled on the edge of a sofa. He wanted to be close to the door.

He is a handsome, healthy looking, 185 pound, 6 feet 1inch tall white male. He describes his symptoms to me: He's nervous all the time, he worries, he paces at home, he's unable to sit still, he's not sleeping, waking up at 4 a.m., having nightmares, constantly looking outside the house through windows, feeling extremely paranoid that his life is in danger, worrying about his wife and a court date next month. He sleeps with a pistol to protect his family. He has a bad temper and yells and screams; he was that way even as a teenager. He's been drinking six to 10 beers every day for the past few months. He is not eating well, and he's lost 10 pounds in two months. He smokes two packs of cigarettes a day. He says he's not using any other drugs or taking over-the-counter medications. He has obsessive-compulsive symptoms of checking, cleaning, washing clothes every day. He's not suicidal, he says, or homicidal. He's never tried to kill himself and doesn't feel manic or have panic disorder symptoms.

Paul says he's had a history of depression since his teen years. He's been paranoid and obsessive-compulsive for five or six years.

Paul is the only child of his biological parents. He was born in Montana, and his family moved to North Carolina when his parents separated; Paul was 4 years old. His mother is 51 years old and she is obsessed with being sick and washing her hands. She has been treated with Zoloft and Prozac. He sees his biological father about once a year.

After high school, Paul got an associate's degree in computer programming. He worked for a local bank for three years in their IT department. He's been unemployed for six months. He has 4-year-old fraternal twins from a previous relationship. They live with their mother in another state, and he pays child support. Paul has been married for less than two years.

His current stressors are the impending court date of being implicated in a drug deal, financial problems, and being unemployed. His wife, parents and stepfather are very supportive.

Based on this information, my diagnostic impression is Major Depressive Disorder, severe, with psychotic features, Generalized Anxiety Disorder, Obsessive Compulsive Disorder,

Nicotine and Alcohol Dependence, and Intermittent Explosive Disorder.

I educate Paul about his psychiatric diagnosis and the rationale of my choice of medications and their side effects. I strongly recommend psychotherapy, and a reduction of alcohol and cigarette smoking. I further caution him about the pistol; he needs to put it in a safe place or give it away. I start him on Remeron, Trazodone and Hydroxyzine.

At the return visit Paul says he's been taking only the Trazodone and Hydroxyzine. He stopped taking Remeron as it made him angry. He's sleeping better, and he's not feeling as paranoid. He has reduced his beer intake from eight to ten cans a day to two or three. He complains that he's getting angrier and has a very short temper. He is quite irritable and depressed. He denies having any suicidal thoughts. I give him samples of Lexapro and Risperdal.

Two weeks later, Paul is smiling more, laughing at times. He is much less paranoid, and hasn't been checking who was outside the house. He's even stopped checking to see if someone is following him in his car. The voice in his head is more positive. He is still sleeping better and isn't worrying as much that the Mafia is going to come and get him. He says he was surprised that when he went to sleep, his pistol was not always under his bed. It was in the other room, and he was not worried. He is also not cleaning as much as he used to do. He's not even drinking every day. He used to start drinking in the morning to take the edge off, but last week he felt confident to go for a job interview and felt good about himself. He has had no side effects from the medications. I increase his Lexapro to 20 mg and continue on Risperdal 1 mg, and Trazodone 50 mg.

A month later, Paul is continuing to improve in his mood, paranoia, obsessions and tempers. He is not hiding himself from the world, and he isn't sleeping with a pistol anymore. His thinking has become clearer, and he feels motivated to look for a job and be successful. He's getting outside the house and talking to more people. His libido is low, and he's still got about 20% residual paranoia. So I increase his Risperdal to 1.5 mg and add Wellbutrin to his medications.

A month later, Paul is making progress. He got a job as a real estate agent and sold one house for over $300,000. He's very happy. He's talking to customers. His sex drive has come back. He feels optimistic and happy about his future life.

AFTER TREATMENT

"I ask myself, is this false hope brought on by medication? I don't know. I feel that the feelings and thoughts I had before were false, but in some way not false at all. Although some of the people I have referred to are very real in this life, I am becoming less concerned about whether or not they're coming to get me. Day by day I am becoming stronger and more confident inside. And I now know that true strength comes from within one's self. I still occasionally look out the window and worry. I know that eventually, someday I will be able

to stop looking over my shoulder. My inner voice has more positive things to say lately, and that is a good thing.

"To describe how I feel after receiving treatment ... is difficult for me to do. To be able to describe a special feeling or emotion would not do it justice. I am today a better and stronger person. Things have seemed to 'smooth out' in my life. The feelings of everyone in the world being out to get me- fade with each passing day. Although I still feel a little paranoid from time to time, I try and take a deep breath and have become able to overcome the feeling. I find myself able to deal with everyday events in a different way than I have dealt with them in the past. I have started to realize that my life is like most people's lives. I have the same problems, whether they be emotional, financial, or just everyday problems that the world has a way of throwing at you. This has become a quality of life I never knew existed, and would have never achieved without help.

"I have a completely new career that I have chosen for myself. Before, I worked for 12 years as a computer engineer for a large company where I could stay buried in my work behind an office door, never dealing with human contact. I have chosen now to sell real estate; I see people all day and constantly communicate with different individuals on a daily basis. I truly believe that this would not have been possible without the help of counseling and medication, and I have no desire to work in an environment that hides me for the outside world ever again.

"If you have read the first part of this story and know the person I was and how I felt, I know you're asking yourself, 'How can this be possible?' I have asked myself that same question and decided

that it's not a question I need to have answered right now. I find positive in all that I do or attempt to do -- whether I fail or succeed, there is a positive lesson learned. This has been a tremendous help in self-growth and purpose in life. After thirty-one years on the planet, I have begun to understand and see things for the first time. ... I notice the color green over all other colors for some reason, and I find it to be a very stimulating color. That may sound a little strange, and I can't explain it myself. ... I do know this: I wake with the feeling of wanting to take on this world, overcome any problem, succeed and move forward in life. ... I have had set backs, as everyone has, but I will not and cannot allow that to hold me down in life any longer. I must move forward, I must succeed in my goals, and I must not be afraid any longer of what I cannot control or change. I must allow myself to live again".

CHAPTER 10

My Twilight Labyrinth by

Howard Brant, D. Miss

Over the past year, I have been on a journey along paths here-to-fore unknown – at least for me. I share my twilight labyrinth in hopes that it may bring encouragement and light to another traveler who may follow along this same path. If by sharing, I can encourage or enlighten –then it will be worth my having traveled it – and sharing this story.

Born in Canada, I was raised as the only child of missionary parents. Growing up in Ethiopia, East Africa, I was close to my family – particularly my father whom I both loved and highly respected.As a boy, I made a personal commitment to become a follower of Jesus Christ.One could call me a "born-again Christian."After finishing high school, I attended a Bible College in Western Canada. There I met my life-long companion and best friend – now my wife of 37 years. Together we have had three wonderful children (and three grandchildren). After finishing our schooling, my beloved and I went to Africa as missionaries – and were there for 12 years between 1971 and 1983. At that end of our time in Africa, we returned to the States and both worked on our post-graduate degrees, she in anthropology and me in the science of mission called "missiology."

As a committed believer, of evangelical Christian belief, I have pastored a church, worked as a missionary, and presently serve as an executive in a large (2000 member) mission organization. In that capacity I travel widely and am deeply involved in Christian activity and ministry.

Late in November 2002, I was on a trip into Ethiopia. Our mission was facing incredible problems – for too complex to record here. But there were situations in both Ethiopia and Sudan that involved personal conflict, disagreements, and my personal intervention. In addition to these problems, I was road weary from crisscrossing time zones, long meetings, and plenty of high tension. Frankly, my mind, emotions and spirit were wearing thin.

As these pressures mounted, I found myself unable to sleep at nights. I'm normally a night owl and work all kinds of strange hours. But this was different. I would lay awake, tossing on my bed all through the night. During those hours, I would simply cry out to my Heavenly Father as did the Lord Jesus when He prayed, "Save me from this hour." On that particular trip I was invited to go away into the mountains of Ethiopia and preach in an area where my wife and I had started a number of Ethiopian (Evangelical) churches many years ago. Though the people there were like my own spiritual children, I simply could not go. I was terribly exhausted. I needed a break – and someone suggested that I take a few days break at a vacation spot reserved for our missionaries in Ethiopia.

While on this little retreat, I found a secluded spot to contemplate what was happening to me. I sat on a large rock by a lake and tried to figure things out.I sat alone for several hours pondering my plight. I just talked to the Lord out loud for hours on end. It was just "stream of conscience" kind of talking. I knew I was on the verge of burnout, breakdown, or whatever you call it. I went to my Bible and tried to discover the root cause of that which seemed to torment my mind. I spent much time studying the Gospels.

As I read, I began to develop a thesis – that the fear (which I was certainly feeling) was directly related to my lack of faith. And faith, it appeared, is often related to a "hardness of heart." This I could not understand – for any "hardness of heart" on my part was not evident to me. Yes, I could think of times I had stepped on peoples toes or thought harshly of people with whom I did not agree. I knew I could quickly dismiss others whom I did not deem informed on the issues that interested me. But "hardness of heart"- I couldn't see it.

In this twilight labyrinth I took a turn -- from bad to worse. When I returned to the States, my own children could see that something was seriously wrong with dad. My eldest confronted me, "Dad, you are going into depression – you need help!" My colleagues at work saw it, too. They encouraged me to get some time off – "completely away from everything." They even changed my e-mail account so that only my secretary could read my mail and she could pass on important items to another on our leadership team. Before I knew it, my beloved and I were on our "break," traveling to Amman, Jordan for Christmas with my daughter and her husband. We were booked to fly on to Bangladesh for more business meetings. My CEO and management team told me plainly, "you don't need to go on to Bangladesh if you don't feel like it."

I remember getting on the airplane at Douglas International Airport in Charlotte, North Carolina. We were on our way to Jordan in the Middle East.This was just prior to the US led war in Iraq. Coming into the airport were about a dozen buses filled with military personnel headed for the impending war in Iraq. As we boarded our plane, I remember thinking, "I will never see this country again."

Christmas in Jordan is a bit of a blur in my mind even now. Even though I was away from my office, my worries followed me. I was losing weight rapidly (about two pounds a day). I could NOT sleep. While I never became irrational – I began seeing potential problems behind everything. As things got worse and worse I imagined problems behind every possible situation. Being in Jordan where the steely eyes of Arabs would look right through me did not help.

Even now it is difficult to put into writing all that went thru my mind in those days. In that time of incredible weakness, my dear one was both tender and strong for me. By then, I had stopped eating solid food because I was sure that I had a bowel obstruction. My wife and daughter felt inside my abdomen and they too could feel "the lump" – which to my mind was nothing short of life threatening cancer. The thoughts that went thru my mind during that period are personal and rather sacred to me. A few months back, I was able to share fully with my dear one – and she and I will keep it between us.

Trip cut short, I found myself back in the doctor's office. Full physical examination. Tests. Depression medication!

We were pretty open with our staff at work – and in one wonderful gesture of love and kindness, they surrounded me, laying hands on me and praying for my recovery. News got out that "something is wrong with Howie."

I was on some sort of depression medication but it was doing nothing for me. Around four AM, I would start to feel hot in bed (we were into winter in the States by this time.) I would throw off the covers and shake the sheet up and down to blow cool air under the covers. By the time to get up, I had a terrible knot in the pit of my stomach.

I began seeing a counselor, and he encouraged me to repeat something from God's Word so as to focus my mind on that, rather than "all my worries." I would sit in our living room sofa. I would rock back and forth because of the painful knot in my stomach. I would wring my hands. I could hear myself panting for air. During these episodes my dear one would hold me tight and we would recite Psalm 23 over and over. "The Lord is my shepherd... He restoreth my soul...Yea though I walk thru the valley of death, I will fear no evil." By this time, I had been thru a number of expensive medical procedures – but all results were negative. At the end of the road I faced the grim possibility that I would have to face a psychiatrist plus a counselor. To my mind at that time – that was the worst possible thing that could happen to me.

I had to wait several weeks for my first appointment -- still sleepless, still panic stricken. In terms of my life experience, I was now caught in a dark labyrinth from which I could see no exit.

I will never forget my trip to the psychiatrist. Unbeknown to those who recommended me to him, this man was of Asian descent and a follower of the Sikh-Hindu Unitarian Universalist faith. Inside his office were models/statues/gods of a religious nature. There sat Buddha next to Christ, next to other Hindu or Buddhist gods.Outside of his office was a category of people I had never "seen" before. They were people just like me who were all torn up inside. I could see it in their faces. I could read it in their eyes. Surely I had not become like one of "these" people.

Dr. Sethi, for that was his name, asked a lot of questions about how I had become this way. I was so ashamed and embarrassed to tell him these things. He asked about all my physical symptoms. As he probed these issues, I suddenly realized that this man had met many people like me before. Diverse in culture, background and religious orientation though we were, I could see that he had mastered the science of the physical mind. I don't remember much about those early meetings except two things. First he told me, "I will get you out of this." Second, he went into his "store room" and brought me three kinds of medications and gave me very strict orders as to how they were to be administered.

Even now, I cannot tell you how all this worked out. All I know is that within two days of starting those medications, my life started to change. I slept for the first time in months – so soundly that my beloved was afraid for me. With the return of sleep, I was sure I had completely recovered – but not Dr. Sethi. He kept me on those meds saying in his wonderful Asian mannerism, "We wouldn't want to have a relapse now, would we?"

As he studied me, I studied him. In some strange way, I became personally attached to this dear man. I came every two weeks at first, then every three, then once a month and now we see each other about once every six weeks or two months.

We would talk about the world of politics and our common interests in Asia. About three quarters of the way thru the discussion, he would casually ask how I was feeling and then write out my prescription for the next session. I learned that his alchemy was in the mixture of drugs he was prescribing for me. He had theories of how one drug combined with another had certain effects. I think he was happy with my progress because the daily cocktail he prescribed for me seemed to be working pretty well.

Even though I thought I was fully cured in just a few weeks, I can see in retrospect that all that had happened was that the meds Dr. Sethi had put me on had stopped my downward spiral. He knew, (and I didn't) that it would take a long while to get those neurons inside my brain cells firing properly again.

During this time, I had the most wonderful support team imaginable. My beloved was always at my side. What can I say? My children surrounded me with love and kindness. I will never forget my 27-year-old son who wept one day as he talked to me. His thesis of life was exactly as mine had been. All things to him had a spiritual root and I must not be trusting God enough. Even though I now hold a slightly different view, I loved his passion, and the fact that he would take on his own dad in such a loving way. Thank you son, I love you for this.

During this whole time, we were quite open about the process with our mission leadership. They never knew how deep this thing went – but they were always most supportive. I offered my resignation to my Director. He would not hear of it – but he did do the very best thing he could possibly have done. That was to allow me to keep coming to work – and do what I could do. He appointed several people to take over parts of my job that were daunting to me. He himself took on the worst problems and always included me in the decisions even though I could only sit there silently and listen.

At work I was still terrified to open my e-mail. Ghosts jumped out on every page. I literally feared to open some files! I would pick out the easy ones – but week-by-week I learned to handle more and more complex issues. At home, I could not look at the TV. Violent scenes and "news of the war" set me off. Even reading the newspaper was a "no-go."

I might just add here, that I had begun seeing a Christian counselor. I'm sure that counselors must have a very important place in the restoration of people like me. But somehow we just didn't connect. I told him so at our second meeting.As I look back now, I should have given him more of a chance. We could have talked more about what got me into this situation and what could be done to prevent anything like this from happening again. But at the time, I sized up the situation thinking that I knew about as much regarding counseling as this man. I knew instinctively which theory of counseling he was following by the types of questions he was asking – and it just didn't work. My true counselors were my friends, my wife, my family, those with whom I work – for they knew my issues and had somehow graciously decided to accept me as I was/am.

Now, all during these many months (for this odyssey took about a year in the telling) something deep was happening inside of me. I had been torn down to rock bottom emotionally, psychologically and spiritually. I forced myself to keep teaching an adult Sunday School class all during this time. Again the class was most supportive. Many of my lessons were wooden and some even harsh. Over the period of a year, the compassion, the tenderness, and perhaps something of the spiritual strength I had once enjoyed began to come back – but slowly – over a period of time.

What was happening to me, however, is that I had walked into a new world. In this labyrinth, I had joined others who had gone thru what is called "burnout" or "breakdown" or "panic attacks" or whatever you want to call it. As I sat in my church one Sunday and I looked down the pew, I saw those who were too weak to stand and others sitting with that same look on their faces as I had on mine. Instinctively I knew them. I could feel their heart. I knew their problem.

One day my wife and I went to a supermarket. There I spotted a young man with a tag attached to his shirt. He limped a little and had a caregiver close beside him. I never would have "seen" people like him before. But now I saw him – and I knew what was going on inside of him. I walked over and gave him a hug! Yes – a big hug! He smiled back so knowingly. Somehow we understood each other.

And that is the way it has been. I can see the hurting now in a new way. Also, in the past few weeks I have seen something for which I am trying to find new categories to understand. Those who know me very well know that even though I am a very public person (that is I do a lot of work publicly) I am rather shy in personal situations. My wife would say that I am a person who does not need a lot of social interaction. While I have confidence to perform well in public, when I am alone on an airplane or on a train, I will just sit quietly and read a book but never engage strangers in conversation – or Christian witness. I have had some concerns about this – but it is a reality of my personality.

Somehow in the past weeks and months, this social reticence has diminished. Now, I feel like I can talk to almost anyone. I recently found myself deeply engaging an Indian economist on the flight over to Ethiopia. In the town shops or along the street – I now have no problem at all talking to complete strangers, and sharing with them some playful chatter or spiritual insight.

Now for a long time, my beloved has been telling me that I must tell my Dr. Sethi that he has to get me off these meds. She and I know that many people in my situation become dependant upon medication.Some people never get off of "mood elevators." I keep telling my wife that I trust this man and he knows best what he is doing.

As I prepared recently for a trip which would take me right around the world, I counted out my meds very carefully. I counted out exactly enough to fill my pillbox – and then enough for each day along the journey. The pillbox has a slot for each day. When I finished the first week of my journey, I went to refill the pillbox – I could not find my medication. Somehow, I had forgotten to put it into my travel bag.At first, I panicked, but then I considered that there was a Doctor higher than Dr. Sethi and He was telling me that my prescribed medication had now come to an end. I was coming out of my twilight labyrinth.For the past three weeks, I have been medication free and feeling on top of the world.

Well, as I write these words, I am back where this all started. I'm back in Ethiopia not far from the very spot where I sat beside the lake and talked to God about my fear, my lack of faith, my hardness of heart. Tomorrow, I will set out on a sort of pilgrimage to that very spot. There I will thank God for allowing me to pass thru the valley of death so that I might learn to see other who walk there as well.I will thank Him for helping me recover from my "hardness of heart." And I will thank Him for "restoring my soul."

The last part of this pilgrimage will take place when I go back to the States and tell my Dr. Sethi a big thank-you for being one thru whom the Heavenly Doctor has worked in my life. I may need dear Dr. Sethi again someday –and if I do, I will not hesitate to ask. But unless I miss my guess, I think he will tell me that I am free to go now – with no prescription this next month.

I still have questions as to my diagnosis. Was my problem spiritual as I thought – or was it a chemical imbalance in my brain? Somehow, I believe that Dr. Sethi and I would agree that there are two sides, maybe three, in all of us. Nothing is just spiritual. Nothing is just physical. These two must be intertwined. Did God heal me – or did Dr. Sethi? I would say BOTH!

Seldom, I believe, does God give his children a clear panoramic view of our own earthly future. Because His eternal purpose is to fashion and mold our faith – it would be contrary to His purpose to tell us what all lies ahead. Despite our strong prayers, God often leaves a cloud around His present workings – and only as we look back upon the path by which we have come, can we see His faithfulness all along the way.

INTERNIST'S REPORT

HB had done an excellent job of controlling his diabetes, blood pressure and elevated cholesterol by diet, exercising and weight loss. He used to take Glucophage (metformin), Atenolol, and Pravachol. Since he came back from Sudan, he has been emotionally upset, not sleeping, loss of appetite and continually second guessing himself. His wife thought that this was just a temporary funk, but it has gone on longer and more severe than she had ever seen.

His physical symptoms included loss of 20 pounds due to lack of appetite, irregular bowel movements, interrupted sleep patterns, blood sugar higher than usual, cold feet, and physical exertion leaving him feeling weak.

His mental/emotional symptoms exhibited a sense of dread as he ponders some of the difficult problems dealing with his job, oversensitivity and worry for people for whom he is responsible, feeling that he may be making bad decisions, and loss of optimism and confidence. His melancholic mood is fluctuating. It comes and goes.

Spiritually, HB finds great comfort in the Psalms. He has been praying more than usual.

He has been productive, coping, and to those who do not know him, he looks fine.

At the urging of his family, HB finally sought help with his doctor.

His physical exam and lab results were unremarkable. Abdominal CT scan and colonoscopy were negative.

A thorough computerized mental health screen indicated difficulty falling asleep, waking often at night, sudden attacks of anxiety or panic attacks, distress over the disorganized way the mind works, can't control thinking the same thoughts over and over, feels apprehensive, worries about a lot of different things, and feels burdened with too many responsibilities.

He was started on Ambien 10 mg as needed for sleep, and Prozac 20 mg a day.

Since there was no significant improvement in over two months, a psychiatric consultation was recommended with Dr. Sethi, along with psychotherapy sessions with a Christian counselor.

PSYCHIATRIC TREATMENT

HB is a congenial friendly 5 feet 11 inches tall, white married male who was accompanied by his wife to my office.

HB described his current symptoms of feeling very anxious, having panic attacks, especially in the morning of sudden onset of shortness of breath, feeling nervous and sweaty, having tingling feelings in feet and hands, with a knot in his abdominal area, and having no appetite, and lost 40 pounds from 246 to 206 pounds in 3 months. Further, he feels hot and cold, and has been worrying a lot. He has been prescribed Ambien for sleep, and Prozac 20 mg that he has been taking for a month from his Internist. There is no significant improvement in his symptoms.

His symptoms started last year in November when he had to make a difficult decision of closing a missionary orphanage in Sudan. HB is Deputy International Director for Asia and East Africa for SIM International. SIM stands for Serving in Mission. Due to not feeling well, he had to cancel his meetings in Thailand, Africa and Bangladesh, for which he feels ashamed and a failure.

There is no previous history of anxiety, panic or depressive symptoms. Also there are no obsessive compulsive symptoms. HB denies any symptoms of paranoia, delusions or hallucinations. He denies abuse of alcohol, drugs, cigarettes or excessive caffeine. He denies any over the counter medications.

On a scale of 1 to 10, 10 being the best and 1 being worst, HB described his functioning at work, home and social settings to be around 1. On the same scale 10 having no symptoms of anxiety or panic attack, and 1 being the worst, he described himself around 1.

HB's mother is 83 year old, and his father died at the age of 74. He is the only child from same parents. His parents were missionaries. There is no history of anxiety, depression, and suicide or alcohol abuse in the family.

He was born in Canada, and raised in Ethiopia. He has a Doctorate in Missiology -- a degree in religion with specialization in missions. He got married at the age of 21 to Joanne his wife, for the past 37 years. He has three children from the ages of 26 to 31, and they are all well settled. He has been working for SIM for 31 years. His current position is the Deputy International Director for Asia and East Africa. Currently he is living in Charlotte for a few years. He has excellent support with his family and friends at SIM. His major stressors are related to his job, namely closing of an orphanage in Sudan that he founded, and his inability to travel for his meetings.

In view of these findings, my diagnosis was Generalized Anxiety Disorder and Panic Disorder without agoraphobic features.

I educated HB and his wife on the psychiatric diagnosis and my rationale of medications and their side effects. He was taken off of Prozac, and started on Paxil, as well as Xanax as needed. He was given samples of Remeron to take at night. A return appointment was given in 2 weeks.

HB reported overall feeling better. His anxiety and panic attacks were better. His appetite had picked up and he gained 4 pounds. His worrying was subsiding, and he was not obsessed about the events in Sudan. The knot in his abdomen was not bothersome. Tingling in his hands and feet was also subsiding. He had started seeing the Christian therapist as well. I continued Paxil CR 25 mg, along with Alprazolam 0.25 mg, and Remeron Sol 15 mg.

At the next session in two weeks, HB was feeling 90% better. He was eating a little too much, and had gained 10 more pounds. His mood and anxiety symptoms were improving. He was sleeping better. He was not as obsessed about his bowel movements as he used to be. He started some teaching and resumed all his responsibilities of work in Charlotte, NC. He was still afraid of traveling overseas. He had an upcoming meeting in Chicago in a month. He felt confident to go to that meeting. His blood sugar and blood pressure were also stabilized, and within normal range. Overall he was happy with the progress. I discontinued Remeron.

I continued to see HB once a month initially and then once in 2 months.

His meeting in Chicago went well. He had another meeting in Ashville where Missionaries from all over the world were coming, and he had to give a big presentation. He handled that stress well. In summer he made a ten days trip to different countries in Africa giving presentations and chairing meetings. He had no problems.

In summer, HB came with his wife, Joanne, to my office. She was happy with the progress. He had no symptoms of anxiety and depression. He felt tired in the day time and started taking a nap. His creativity was not as it used to be, and his sexual desire was also decreased. In view of this I reduced Paxil to 15 mg, and advised him to take Alprazolam as needed.

HB resumed his hectic life of travel to Africa and Asia. He felt very happy to be able to function at his best capacity. His creativity came back and he had no side effects from the medications. He was surprised that his social anxiety had decreased significantly, and he was able to talk to strangers without feeling shy or embarrassed.

At his last visit in December 2003, he forgot to take his medications with him to his trip to Ethiopia, Thailand, Korea and Japan. He had not taken his medication for over 2 weeks, and he felt very good. He expressed his desire to go off the medications altogether, to which I gladly agreed. I cautioned him, however, to resume them should any of the symptoms come back, and come for an early appointment to see me.

Chapter 11

A Psychiatrist's Story

"Physician heals thyself". How often those words have rung in my ears. Mostly others were kind enough not to say them, but my own superego bombarded me with them.

I was blessed with a high IQ. But from the beginning, life was difficult for me. My mother told me, when I was a baby, it seemed she couldn't manage three children. My guess is that she had a postpartum depression; but she was not depressed thereafter, despite having two more children, and being married to a severely depressed man who also had a problem with rage and alcohol.

The apple falls close to the tree. Of my parents five children, I am by far the most like my father. He had long periods of depression with sadness, withdrawal and loss of functioning. He was hospitalized on several occasions and had electroshock therapy on three different occasions. He was morose and disabled most of his adult life. He died at the age of 58 in a mental hospital.

So I used to say that I went to psychiatry to cure my father--symbolically, of course. But the old saying that psychiatrists are trying to solve their own problems was partly true for me. I was a miserable adolescent, excluded from the "in" crowd and tormented by longing for a girl who did not return the favor. But I was the smart one who won a scholarship to Harvard.

Talk about culture shock: from a small mill town in the South to the center of learning in the North. It was a feast for the intellect, but with my natural shyness, I was in over my head socially.

I stuck it out, studied hard and got good grades. But in my senior year, I became unable to study. I could not concentrate. I went to the college psychiatrist and got some amphetamines, which seemed to help. I think I was depressed and fearful of moving on to unfamiliar territory. The same thing happened in my senior year of medical school at Duke University. I saw the psychiatrist again and muddled through.

I have been taking antidepressant medication for so long I cannot remember when I began. I took Tofranil, then Pamelor, and they seemed to help. But when my first marriage ended in divorce, I plunged into a severe depression that lasted eight months.

I showed up for work each day at the hospital, but I could barely function. Again I entered psychotherapy and it helped me to weather the storm and get back on my feet.

Life was more enjoyable for a while. I had a midlife fling and drank a lot of alcohol and experimented with cocaine and marijuana. I had conflicts with colleagues and nurses, but otherwise life was good.

I entered solo private practice and built up a thriving hospital practice by allying myself with mental health centers in the area. They referred me patients who needed hospital admission and who had some means to pay for private care.

I was riding high. I worked up to 14 hours a day (at the age of 50) and made lots of money.

Then, came the fall. The hospital authorities called me into a meeting and threatened to revoke my hospital privileges. They said I had offended nearly every nurse in the department of Psychiatry. Moreover, nurses reported that I could not remember my patients and that I sounded strange on the telephone at night. The authorities decided that I needed a leave of absence and a substance abuse evaluation.

I went to a substance abuse treatment center for 28 days. I've not had a drop of alcohol nor any illegal drug since then for more than 15 years. I saw a distinguished psychiatrist who told me I had a Bipolar Disorder and started me on Lithium Carbonate that I have taken ever since.

But my practice crumbled and my second wife sued for divorce and my colleagues shunned me. I fell into another spell of severe depression.

Since then I have had nine jobs. I was an excellent diagnostician and prescriber of psychiatric medications, but angry rages and depression led to conflicts with the staff and patients. For the last five years I haven't been able to hold a job for more than eight months.

What angers me most is being treated with disrespect. When I began my Residency training at UCLA, the doctor was an admired and respected member of the community. He hung out a shingle and seldom moved. His career and financial security were assured. His professional judgment was seldom questioned.

None of the above is true any more, at least, not for me. I find many young doctors brash, demanding and disrespectful. Times have changed and I have been unable to make the adjustment.

Many people have helped me along the way, such as the psychiatrist who realized I was Bipolar, members of my support group, especially my sponsor of the last five years. My wife has been loyal and supportive.

I have a severe Bipolar disorder but I do fairly well. I no longer try to practice psychiatry. I occupy myself at baby sitting my grandson for several hours each day. I enjoy him immensely. He is a gift from Heaven.

In the old Freudian way of thinking, people were sick because of bad experiences, bad thoughts and bad decisions. I believe that because I am ill I have had bad experiences and thoughts, and made bad decisions.

Thank God that now-a-days there are good numbers of mood stabilizing medications and antidepressants. I regret that I could not bring my intellectual gifts to bear for the benefit of myself and others. But I remind myself: I didn't ask for this disease and I didn't cause it. God willing I will sometimes be able to rise above it.

SECTION TWO :

ASSORTED STORIES

As you sow, so shall you reap; this body is the result of your actions.

Sikhism

Hatred breeds confusion. Clear thinking and careful action can come only when the heart is free from hatred.

Gita

To a mind that is "still" the whole universe surrenders.

Taoism

The peacemakers, and not the warmakers, are blessed. Those who take the sword shall perish by the sword. War is the road to destruction, while peace is the road to happiness and prosperity.

Christianity

Meditate upon God and you will find peace. Meditation must be in humility and constant if one would achieve its true reward.

Islam

The wise man is slow to wrath. He gives soft answers and thereby turns away wrath on the part of others. Love, and not wrath, should be the goal of true believers, for wrath leads to strife.

Judaism

CHAPTER 12

Introduction

There are limits to what writers can tell readers and artists can tell viewers. Perhaps he is Lancelot with the world and his life in ruins around him, but there is a prospect of a new world in the Shenandoah Valley. There was something wrong with the old world, the old things, the old flowers, the old skies, old clouds— or something wrong with his way of seeing them. They were used up. They have to be seen anew. Here is a new sky, a new sea, a new rose . . .

Walker Percy

One of the most startling realizations is to see ourselves as others do. It is like hearing your recorded voice, or accidentally catching your reflection in a mirror, thinking it was someone else.

Listening to my patients' stories, I realized there are limits to what we can tell others about ourselves, and that the mystery of healing must also be recorded from the outside. Physician's charts and hospital records are usually one dimensional, but when seen against a patient's own voice, they lend depth and perspective. Like a three-way mirror, they allow a glimpse of ourselves as others may see us. So in Section II of this book, I've included my own perspective of other patients seen through my office notes.

There was something wrong in these people's world, or at least something distorted in the way they perceived it.How do we move from an old world with old things that use us up into seeing things anew—"a new sky, a new sea, a new rose?"Indeed, it is an incredible journey.

These are stories from the hill that I stand on, the one we call psychiatry. There are limits here, too, but the view has been endlessly fascinating.Views of an addict who took his own life, a physician's addiction and bipolar illness, stories of the inscrutable enigma of sexuality, a patients paranoid delusion disorder probably misdiagnosed for 40 years as schizophrenia. It is talking to a person caught in the endless cycles of an Obsessive Compulsive Disorder, plucking their hair a strand at a time, or taking endless . notes always wishing they could just stop. Seeing a person so close to killing themselves, then with the help of medication and therapy, recovering and taking charge of their lives is to be part of an art that is wondrous. As a person hears their own history and realizes their illnesses is not the result of abuse or something they did, but rather from sheer genetics, scales fall from the eyes, and people humbly stand and get on with life.

Listen, empathize, shed tears, and be grateful to those patients and researchers who have seen anew so others need not forever retrace their painful steps!

CHAPTER 13

Death By Suicide

The fear that kills;
And hope that is unwilling to be fed;
Cold, pain, and labour, and all fleshy ills;
And mighty Poets in their misery dead.
--Perplexed, and longing to be comforted,
my question eagerly I did renew.
'How is it that you live, and what is it you do?'

William Wordsworth

Ruth was 53 when she first came to see me, a blonde, blue-eyed very attractive German American who spoke English with a German accent. She was elegantly dressed and groomed meticulously. She was accompanied by her husband, Heinz. She was 5 feet, 5 inches tall and weighed 135 pounds. She had been seeing a female therapist for several years when her OB/GYN recommended recently that she see a psychiatrist.

She came to her first session in the spring of 1999. She was vague about her history, but Heinz said she'd had a history of depression for at least six years, and that she had taken Prozac for a year but had become nervous and anxious. On a visit to Munich, Germany, to see family, she had become delusional and paranoid with suicidal thoughts, and thus was hospitalized for four weeks. She was given a diagnosis of Schizoaffective Disorder and was initially treated with Stelazine and then Risperdal and Amitriptyline, which caused her to gain weight and suffer dry mouth.

Ruth made it clear that she did not like treatment with "chemicals," that she did not trust Western medicine or pharmaceutical companies. She liked herbal therapy and had tried St. John's Wort for several months, though it did not help. She believed strongly in herbal teas, "natural healing," massage therapy and Yoga. She was an avid Yoga practitioner and meditated daily for 30 to 40 minutes. She was a vegetarian who believed in the power of mind over body and spirit, and had read all books from Dr. Deepak Chopra. She had even gone to several Yoga Ashrams in the United States and in India to spiritually purify her body and mind. She believed in peace and the power of love to solve world problems.

One of the primary reasons Ruth was so scared of Western medicines was that her mother had committed suicide at the age of 54 by overdosing on prescription drugs. She was afraid that she had the same illness as her mother, and did not want to become like her. So she began to seek her answers in Eastern medicine and philosophy.

She had very clear thoughts but was curious about why she couldn't control her emotions or thoughts. She exhibited paranoia, saying that she was scared that someone was watching her most of the time. She checked her doors frequently to make sure they were locked. She also saw images of different Indian gods and even Jesus Christ talking to her.

Ruth looked healthy but was very sad. She had stopped drinking wine and had begun to refrain from making love to her husband. Heinz said her mind was always "preoccupied," and agreed that she avoided intimacy. He also said that there were times Ruth had "an odd look" about her that frightened him and their children.

She was no longer able to function at home, feeling sad but unable to cry. She felt disconnected, had few friends, and did not like "being herself." She was no longer able to focus enough to read or work; she saw herself as detached, apart from life itself. Yet she denied being suicidal.

Except for suffering the negative effects of menopause, Ruth had no medical problems. She did not drink, smoke or abuse drugs. There were no known allergies to medications.

Ruth's father died when he was 70. She has an older brother but is not close to him. He worked in a factory all his life and used to drink heavily. He is now retired.

Despite her mother's suicide, Ruth said she was not aware of any other history of depression, schizophrenia or suicide in the family. All her relatives on both sides of the family died in World War Two.

Ruth was born in Jena, Germany after the war had ended. She completed her middle school and worked in retail. She met her husband, Heinz, when they were children. They immigrated to the United States in 1970. Heinz did his post-doctoral work at prestigious places, and finally accepted the Chair of Physics and Computer Sciences at a university. Ruth was not active in the local German community and became a homemaker. They had very bright children: Elizabeth, 30, an attorney from Harvard Law School who worked in Washington, D.C., and Max, 25, who worked with IBM in Charlotte as a computer research scientist.

Ruth described her stressors as Elizabeth not being married, and her own marital conflict. However, she counted on Heinz for being her support along with a few friends. She listed her strengths as being in good health, educated, and financially secure.

My diagnosis was Major Depressive Disorder with psychotic features. I educated Ruth and Heinz about the seriousness of her illness and about how critical it was that she took her medications as directed. I also cautioned about the genetics of our brain chemistries and thus our behavior and emotions. I was also quite blunt in discussing the susceptibility of suicide in the family. I discontinued her Amitriptyline, started her on Effexor and increased the dose of Risperdal to 1.5 mg at night. I further emphasized a verbal "No Harm" contract, and a return appointment was scheduled for 7 to 10 days.

At the beginning of her second session, Heinz asked to speak to me alone. Ruth said it was OK. He told me that she has suffered from paranoia and depression for at least 25 to 30 years, especially after the birth of their daughter. At that time Ruth had gone into a deep depression and was hospitalized. Heinz said her paranoia included unfounded worries that he was having an affair. She became especially concerned when he attended professional meetings. Her fears caused her to screen all his financial statements. She was additionally fearful that someone was going to harm the children, and that he did not feel comfortable leaving her alone. This information helped to confirm my own diagnosis.

Later in the session, Ruth confirmed that Heinz's statements were true. She appeared less depressed and smiled a bit. She was tolerating the medications without side effects except for mild anxiety during the day. When I prescribed increasing Effexor to 75 mg and Risperdal to 2 mg, and adding a low dose of Alprazolam to take as needed, Ruth objected, saying "I don't want another pill, I hate foreign chemicals going into my pure body." I reminded her the role of medications in her illness. But she was stubborn, saying she only wanted one pill. She asked about homeopathy and a miracle cure with diluted dosages of medications – what did I think of that, and why is it so popular in India?

I told her my honest opinion that the scientific method of clinical testing had not substantiated the theories or the practice of homeopathy. My words did little to dispel her fears or change her opinion.

When I saw her at her next appointment in three weeks, Ruth said she was "cured and didn't need any medications." She had taken the prescriptions for seven days, and then reduced the dosages to one half for a week, then discontinued taking any medications for the past 10 days. She was happy and smiling, saying her paranoia had diminished, and that she had seen a Chinese nature doctor who gave her herbs and recommended massage therapy. Ruth was convinced that Dr. Wong's herbs helped her more than my medications. I cautioned her again about the seriousness of her mental illness. I didn't dismiss her for noncompliance; instead, I asked her to call my office should her situation become worse.

I didn't see Ruth for several months. She had a good summer, but her situation started to deteriorate in the fall. She went to see another psychiatrist who essentially gave her the same diagnosis that I had. He had recommended treatment with antipsychotic and antidepressant medications, saying that if she didn't respond to the medications or if suicidal thoughts became uncontrollable, she should consider hospitalization and electro-shock therapy. She had been taking Zyprexa and Remeron for three months.

The next spring, Ruth came to see me with Heinz. She had gained 20 pounds and felt miserable about it. Her mood and paranoia were better, but she was not able to fit into her clothes, had no desire to exercise, and felt "fat and ugly" at 155 pounds. She craved sweets and ice cream and lost control of her food intake. I gradually reduced the dose of Zyprexa from 10 mg to 2.5 mg, and substituted Remeron with Serzone during the next 30 days. She tolerated these changes well and started to lose weight. Her symptoms were well under control with these medications, and she started to do exercise and her daily routine of Yoga and massage therapy. Once again, she said she distrusted Western medicine and pharmaceutical companies.

Ruth read a book by psychiatrist Peter R. Breggin, M.D., called "Toxic Psychiatry" (1991, St. Martin's Press, New York). Based upon the central theme that therapy, empathy, and love must replace drugs, electroshock, and biochemical theories of the new psychiatry, she started seeing a new therapist who agreed with the premise and did not believe in pharmaceuticals. So she gradually got herself off of all medications. She came to my office in June 2000 with the copy of the book, and challenged me with countless questions.

I was alarmed by Ruth's state of mind and the course she was taking. I asked her to bring her husband to the next visit.

Three weeks later, Ruth showed up with Heinz and Max. Ruth had no objection to them being in the session. I educated them again on Ruth's psychiatric history, her illness and its treatment with medications. I further emphasized the grave possibility of suicide in a most frank and honest way. They questioned me about Dr. Breggin's book and wanted to know how it could be published if he was not right. I emphasized that this is a free country, and there is a freedom of the press.

Ruth was obviously perplexed and felt torn between the two psychiatrists she'd seen and Dr. Breggin's claim that the pharmaceuticals we were prescribing were toxic. Her symptoms of depression and paranoia had begun to resurface. I gave her sample packages of Risperdal and Serzone.

About two weeks later, Heinz called and said that Ruth wasn't taking her medications and her symptoms were deteriorating. We scheduled an appointment at the earliest possible time in three days. When they arrived, Ruth was disheveled and unkempt. She was not eating or sleeping well, awaking several times a night. The paranoia was becoming worse; she was checking the basement and doors so often she was unable to function.

Ruth's mood was very sad, and while she denied any " plans or intent" to kill herself, she admitted fleeting thoughts of suicide. However, Heinz quickly said Ruth had been asking for a rope and had actually gone to Wal-Mart to look for one. I was obviously alarmed, and shared my concern. I strongly recommended immediate resumption of medications, and hospitalization should the situation deteriorate further. I gave them the telephone numbers of the local psychiatric hospitals. I also explained Intensive Outpatient Therapy. Further, I told Ruth and Heinz that the criteria of whether a patient is admitted to the hospital by their HMO are what the patient tells the assessment person. Specifically, a patient will not be authorized for an admission unless the person says that he/she is in danger of "harming self or others."

Ruth was utterly opposed to hospitalization, so I also advised them of the procedure for involuntary commitment to a hospital. We scheduled an appointment within a week, and I strongly recommended she resume therapy as soon as possible.

Two days later, I received a phone call from Max. He said his mother hung herself in the attic. He had found her body and called 911.

I was shocked and angry. I gave Max and Heinz my home and cell numbers so they could contact me any time. After seeing my last patient that day, my wife and I went to their home. We spoke to the family and friends. Heinz said that Ruth awoke early in the morning, made breakfast and appeared less depressed. She was rather affectionate. She was dressed up unusually well with make up, as if she were saying good bye. Heinz felt terribly guilty, repeating that he should have paid closer attention and that he did not give enough care.

Throughout the week, I was numb, and sad. I did not express my feelings to anyone except my wife. I thought of calling one of my psychiatrist friends, but I was afraid to admit that I was unable to save Ruth's life. I did not want to be seen as a failure. This was my first case of completed suicide.

I had been a leader in the community, and I took pride in knowing everything possible in contemporary psychiatry. I often thought that had I been doing inpatient hospital work, I would have fought with the insurance company to have Ruth admitted to a safe place in the hospital and, with the help of medications, perhaps I could have saved her life.

My wife and I went to Ruth's funeral. I was introduced to her family and friends as "Ruth's psychiatrist." I spoke German to the family and friends, giving condolences, and offering help.

COMING TO TERMS

There is a saying in the field, "There are two kinds of psychiatrists: those who have had a patient commit suicide, and those who were waiting for that to happen." During the first 10 years of my practice, I had belonged to the latter; now I was on the other side.

We live and die in a litigious society, and I finally admitted to myself that I had always been worried about a wrongful death lawsuit. It was one of the reasons why I never talked to colleagues about my feelings about Ruth's death. You never know who might be called to testify. In retelling Ruth's story, my story, I realized that I need to come to terms by putting my feelings and reactions on the written page. Perhaps attorneys and forensic psychiatrists would know I tried my best to save Ruth's life. If most of the psychiatric hospitals in this area had not been closed due to systematic defunding by Managed Care, and had I still been doing hospital psychiatry, I may have had a chance of saving Ruth's life. But under the circumstances, I have to conclude that I could not have prevented this tragedy.

Most wrongful death lawsuits are settled out of court. Psychiatrists go through a period of anxiety, depression, a sense of failure, humiliation, worries, sleepless nights, loss of productivity and income. In addition, they suffer an increase in their malpractice premiums, and they are excluded from insurance company panels. Often this all leads to a loss of confidence and the breakup of marriage and relationships. Some never recover from the trauma and continue to exhibit symptoms of post-traumatic stress disorder.

Because of this fear, some psychiatrists and therapists in this area have stopped taking care of patients who have attempted suicide or who have ever been hospitalized. If all psychiatrists and therapists followed this example, then moderately to severely ill patients would have no place to go. Further, I am not sure whether it is ethically or morally right to refuse to treat suicidal patients. Among physicians, psychiatrists are the only ones who are adequately trained to treat patients at risk of suicide.

Likewise, if insurance companies only want patients with low risks, who will take care of high-risk patients? Recently a patient told me that she was paying $440 per month under her COBRA insurance. At the time of renewal of her policy, the agent quoted $2,800 per month. That's $33,600 per year after tax just for health insurance! This patient makes only $10.50 an hour -- or $21,840 yearly before taxes -- at a department store as a beauty and fashion specialist. This is outrageous. I advised her to write to the Insurance Commission, her senators, the governor, and the newspapers.

Most people have no idea doctors are performing under such stress and fear of the lawsuits. Medicine is not a perfect science. It is an art. Society has very high expectations of its doctors. People do not realize that everyone's genetic makeup is unique, and thus their response to medications or surgery is unpredictable. Most doctors would never do intentional harm, yet they are held liable to the highest standards. No other professionals -- lawyers, business people, bankers, financial advisors, or politicians -- are expected to come even halfway to that mark.

And there is a grave crisis in medicine of skyrocketing malpractice premiums for doctors. An OB/GYN has to pay $ 100,000 per year for malpractice insurance in some states. Insurance premiums for even low risk medical specialties have risen three times over the past few years. This is totally out of proportion with their earnings. As a consequence many doctors are deciding not to carry any insurance and go bare, and thus not see patients in the hospitals nor from HMO's who require that physicians on their panel must carry insurance.

Unless these crises are resolved urgently, our best medical system in the world may not remain at its best.

CHAPTER 14

Landlord's Daughter

At the bottom of the heart of every human being,
from earliest infancy until the tomb,
there is something that goes on indomitably
expecting,
in the teeth of all experience
of crimes committed, suffered, and witnessed,
that good and not evil will be done.

Simone Weil

Like miracles, tragedies most often begin in a flash of time. Susan was 17-years-old, a High School Junior, when she walked into a different and unforgiving world. Like a person waking up blind, Susan awoke afraid and depressed. Her stepmother took her to a psychiatrist who treated her with Mellaril and Amitriptyline four times a day, a prescription she took every day for the next 30 years. While Susan remained unaware of her diagnosis, the prescription she was taking was probably for schizophrenia.

When her physician retired, she went to a new psychiatrist who was trained in psychoanalysis. He encouraged her to go off all medications and be treated with psychotherapy alone.

A few years later, the psychotherapist Susan was seeing referred her to my office. When we met, she had not taken the

Mellaril for more than four years. Her primary care physician had prescribed her Amitriptyline.

She said, "I feel imprisoned in my own thoughts." She was continually replaying tapes of trivial and bad things from her past, saying she felt people were "playing with my mind."

Despite more than 30 years of medication and therapy, Susan still suffered from paranoia she had since she was a young girl. Untrusting, she was afraid "of them" and was bothered by crowds and did not like going to parties. Susan said she was eating and sleeping well and had not experienced any crying episodes.Susan did not have any suicidal thoughts and said she did not have any obsessive-compulsive behaviors other than the unremitting paranoia.

At our first session, she was well dressed and groomed, but she appeared older than her age. She had a slight involuntary movement of her lips and tongue that may have been a side effect from 30 years of Mellaril. Her facial expressions were odd, and she was clearly nervous.Susan was working with a well-known insurance company and said she was stressed primarily because she could not focus in her work.

In a few months, Susan was a new person. She would become a woman who not only didn't worry about what others thought of her, but who prevailed through trauma and pain.

She was born in Charleston, South Carolina where her father served in the Navy. Several years later, her mother became pregnant by another man while her father was on tour.Possibly suffering from a mental illness and stressed by her situation,

Susan's mother committed suicide. The family soon moved to Charlotte when Susan was four-years-old.

She graduated from High School and finished one year of secretarial college. In her early twenties, Susan overdosed twice on her medication and was placed in a state hospital for six months. At 39, she married Mark who was 50 and had two adult children from a previous marriage.

Mark had a long history of alcoholism. Susan's sister did not work because of anxiety and panic attacks. In addition, her sister's son, Susan's nephew, suffers from paranoia and delusions.

At 81, Susan's father was retired, previously owning a small insurance company and several buildings in the area. As a successful landlord, he and Susan's stepmother lived in an exclusive retirement community.

Susan said her major stresses included her job and her illness. She received support from her parents, her husband and her Alanon friends (a support group for those with an alcoholic family member or friend). Her strengths included good physical health, a job she enjoyed, and a sharp intelligence.

I diagnosed Susan with Paranoid Delusional Disorder, not Schizophrenia, which was her likely diagnosis when she was 17. I educated her about her condition and the side effects of her medications. I continued her current prescription of Amitriptyline, and added Haloperidol 1 mg at night.

Within two weeks, Susan was an utterly different person. She was feeling better about all aspects of her life, and for the first time in her adult life she felt at peace, saying, "I am finally able to stop repeating the tapes in my mind." As the paranoia lessened, ordinary tasks like going to the grocery store were no longer a frightening journey. She began to feel comfortable with people and actually enjoyed going to parties. She began cleaning her apartment, as she felt less tired and more energetic in contrast to the 30 years of weariness when she had taken Mellaril. As her mental concentration sharpened, Susan became happier and said she was not experiencing any side affects. I discontinued the Amitriptyline and increased the dosage of Haloperidol to 1.5 mg.

Two weeks later, Susan continued to improve. Able to think clearly on her feet for the first time, she went to a company picnic and was able to enjoy the event. Susan was not feeling sleepy during the day, was able to go to shopping malls, and did not feel as though people were staring at her. Her husband also noticed a significant improvement. I recommended that Susan continue the Haloperidol at 1.5 mg for another two weeks and then reduce it to 1 mg and maintain that dosage. A return appointment was scheduled in five weeks.

At her next visit, Susan said she felt good. "It feels almost too good to be true; it's like a dream. I'm able to read, clean house; Mark and I went on vacation and I enjoyed meeting and talking to new people." Clearly, Susan felt more confident as she began to trust her own thoughts. At ease with herself, she no longer felt guilty about herself or her past. She was learning how to live and take joy in the moment, without the paranoid thoughts recurring through her mind. Small concerns were no longer insurmountable, and she quit worrying when Mark spoke to strangers. They enjoyed being together and began making love more often. Susan felt more comfortable at work, and felt at ease when she returned to Alanon meetings.

Two months, later, Susan was feeling proud of her renewed relationship with her father and stepmother who were both hospitalized. She felt coherent and logical and wasn't frightened or disoriented when she visited the hospital. Her thoughts were more coherent and logical, and Susan's parents were proud of her progress and appreciative of her help. At work, she felt progressively more at ease—joking and kidding with others.

We Cannot Control the World

"I can't believe a small pill could change my life after so many years of worries and pain. For the first time I feel like myself, the person I was meant to be." Yet despite the remarkable improvements in her mental health, Susan soon learned to deal with a world she could not control.

I recommended to Susan that she continue working with a therapist to come to terms with her past, the new changes she was going through, and her parents' deteriorating health. Her stepmother died the following January. It was very difficult on her father, as they had been married for 47 years.Susan took a week off from work as she passed through a healthy grieving process.

Later, she enjoyed herself at a family wedding and continued to progress in her work, social, and family situations.

She received good job reviews and had a good professional relationship with her supervisor. Susan continued to support her ill father who gave her a significant monetary gift and discussed the final distribution of his estate. Their relationship continued to improve as Susan visited him twice a week.

She said she felt like a "free person," as she began exploring her own identity. Susan noticed a healthier connection between her thoughts and feelings. With the help of a nicotine patch, she quit smoking, and in the spring was able to tell her life's story to her Alanon group. All these were things she never could have done a year earlier. Susan also began traveling to new places.

Then, like many of us, Susan was forced to deal with several difficult issues at the same time. Her husband Mark developed bone cancer at the same time she lost her job.Though her severance pay ended in a few weeks, she felt confident that she would be able to cope with the situation.

Susan's father began to recover and started seeing another woman he met at the nursing home. Several months after she lost her job, Susan began working for another insurance company as an hourly temporary employee. Her father was planning to remarry despite fracturing his hip and suffering a mild stroke.

Susan was handling all these stressors quite well, but when her sister developed breast cancer, Susan, understandably, began to feel depressed. As the only healthy person in the family, Susan worried she would not be able to cope with the increasing stress of caring for others. In response, I began her on Zoloft 25 mg per day.

Her job became permanent and she received good insurance.Susan's father appointed her the role of durable power of attorney.Feeling his confidence in her, Susan's own self-confidence continued to strengthen. Within six months, she earned two raises and continued to do well in all areas of her life. Her father married after the holidays. Enjoying her new life, Susan hosted a party for the newly weds.

A year later, Susan developed breast cancer and chose to have a lumpectomy. Her father was growing weaker and now had difficulty walking, while her husband Mark was attending a pain center at a local hospital for his own cancer. Not an easy time for anyone, but Susan was dealing with these stressors.

Her father died the following winter; Susan managed the loss and the task of managing the funeral and estate arrangements. Upon receiving half of her father's estate, Mark's children began pressing her for money. She not only endured these additional burdens, but she also passed her insurance exams and continued earning promotions at work.

I had been discussing with Susan a possible change from Haloperidol to newer second generation antipsychotic medications. She tried Risperdal for a month, but her paranoid symptoms started to return. A year later, she tried Geodone, but became lethargic and suffered body aches.

Susan began exercising regularly, walking two miles a day. She visited her sister in Florida and traveled to Boston as she prepared for another promotion. Susan's sister died of a stroke and heart attack at the age of 66. Overall, Susan coped well with the deaths of her stepmother, father, sister, as well as other major stressors. She continues to be emotionally stable, effective at work and comfortable in social settings. Susan continues to take low dosages of Haloperidol and Zoloft, and we have a scheduled appointment every three months.

CHAPTER 15

A Case of Delirium

Anyone who isn't confused doesn't really understand the situation.

Edward R. Murrow

When Maggie and I first spoke, she was extremely nervous and unable to sit still. Pacing constantly in the small room, she was visibly confused and disoriented. She did not know the date, the year, or city she was living in, or the name of the hospital in which we spoke.Her world was bafflement; she had no concept of a history or a coherent present. Her birthday, Social Security number, and former presidents were equal unknowns. Maggie, however, did know her husband's name. Additionally, she was obsessed with family members who died during the past several years—a sister, her mother, and father.

Maggie was 60 years old, and was brought to the psychiatric hospital by Richard, her husband of 40 years. She suddenly became confused and disoriented after a seizure-like episode.Yelling and violent, she was taken to a hospital where general physical tests—CT Brain scan, EEG, EKG, and other lab tests—all were negative. She was released to the care of her primary care physician. He prescribed a sleeping medication, which proved unhelpful.

After she became increasingly confused and disoriented, Maggie was referred to a psychiatric hospital and assigned to my care. As she never had displayed similar symptoms, this was her first stay in a psychiatric hospital.

Born and raised in a rural community, Maggie graduated from High School and completed two years of community college. She married at 20 and worked as a dental assistant and as a clerk in retail stores. She and Richard, who retired from the Railway Services, have a 39-year-old son and a four-year-old grandson.

Both of Maggie's parents are deceased; her mother died of Alzheimer's dementia. She lost her sister a year before from a heart attack, and her brother died of pancreatic cancer when he was only 28. Her stressors included these anniversaries of her relatives' deaths and a conflict with her pastor.

Maggie's family and husband were supportive throughout her treatment.

A through physical examination and blood chemistry tests were preformed: urinalysis, lumbar fluid, HIV test, blood folic acid, and vitamin B-12 levels. They were all negative or within normal ranges. An EEG indicated no epileptic seizures, and an MRI of the brain did not reveal any abnormality. The neurologist's report indicated delirium and dementia, which was consistent with my diagnosis.

For her own safety, an aid was assigned initially to be with Maggie all the time. She was treated with Haloperidol and Lorazepam. The dosages of Haloperidol were titrated up gradually up to 10 mg per day. Lorazepam helped with her agitation and anxiety, and Maggie was given a sleeping pill as needed. She was also prescribed a trial of Risperdal for a week, to which she did not respond.

Richard came daily to the hospital, arriving in the morning and leaving only in the late evening. He and the family were very supportive.

It took almost 15 days for Maggie's symptoms of delirium to clear and memory to improve. She responded well to 5 mg of Haloperidol, and at 2 mg her symptoms recurred.

After three weeks in the psychiatric hospital, Maggie was released and prescribed the following medications: Haloperidol 5 mg at night, Lorazepam 0.5 mg twice daily, and Benztropin 1 mg daily to counter the side effects of Haloperidol. We scheduled an appointment for my office in one week.

It generally requires higher dosages of medications to control symptoms in acute settings such as a hospitalization than in an outpatient setting.Therefore, I was not surprised when Maggie came to my office and she said she was feeling tired and groggy during the day. While her speech was a bit slurred, her memory was good, and she was no longer confused. She knew the day, date, month and year, as well as current events. Her appetite was normal and she was sleeping well. I discontinued the Lorazepam and gradually reduced the Haloperidol from 5 to 3 mg.

Maggie's memory and physical strength improved, and she was able to do her ordinary activities of cleaning, cooking, shopping, and going out to eat with Richard. In response, her dosage of Haloperidol was decreased to 1 mg over the next three months.

Christmas, the New Year, and spring passed well with family and social activities. She resumed her hobby of crossword puzzles and said she felt "100% better." Encouraged by her progress, I reduced her Haloperidol to 0.5 mg during April, and then discontinued it the following month while monitoring her progress.

At the end of September, I received a call from Richard who said Maggie suffered another seizure and had been hospitalized for two days under the care of a neurologist. Numerous additional tests discovered an aneurysm (a dangerous widening of the wall of a blood-vessel, usually an artery) in her brain. She was started on Dilantin—an anti-seizure medication—and Haloperidol. Once again, Maggie was extremely confused and was having difficulty sleeping.

Her symptoms were quite similar to the ones she experienced almost a year before. She was confused with memory loss, and was not aware of her surroundings. Richard said she had been yelling, demanding to go back to the fields so she could pick cotton. I immediately recommended hospitalization.

Remarkably, once again, her disorientation coincided with the anniversaries of the same family members' deaths.The similarity of her psychological symptoms surrounding these anniversaries appeared more than coincidental.

As she responded well to Haloperidol and Lorazepam, these medications were prescribed again along with Prozac to treat her depressive symptoms.Higher dosages of Haloperidol were required during her second hospitalization in order to control Maggie's symptoms of delirium. Once stabilized, she was transferred to the outpatient program where Richard brought her for daily therapy, individual and group sessions.She was eventually discharged on the following medications: Haloperidol 6 mg, Trazodone 100 mg to help her sleep, Lorazepam 0.5 mg three to four times a day, Benztropine 1 mg twice daily to counter the side effects of Haloperidol, Prozac 20 mg, and Dilantin for seizures.

Once she was home, Maggie adjusted well as she returned to her normal activities including shopping. While her mood was improving, and her personality was returning, Maggie complained of memory difficulties. Her neurologist increased her Dilantin, and I reduced the Haloperidol gradually to 4 mg.

At the next visit in two weeks, she had started working on crossword puzzles, but she noticed that she was not as "sharp" as she used to be. Maggie also noted mild drowsiness and tiredness during the day. In response, I reduced the dosages of Haloperidol, Lorazepam, and Benztropin.Four weeks later, Maggie reported no side effects from the medications, saying she had "no complaint" about her memory and her day-to-day functioning was improving.

In the meanwhile, she consulted a neurosurgeon. After an arteriogram of the brain, a surgery was scheduled within a few weeks to remove the aneurism, which was located close to the speech center.

Maggie spent six days in the hospital following a successful surgery in mid-December. She had some initial speech difficulties that improved with time. She was stabilized at Haloperidol 2 mg, Prozac 10 mg, and Lorazepam 0.5 mg twice daily. Her confusion, paranoia, and memory symptoms had dissipated.

The following April, Maggie had another seizure, and was hospitalized briefly. Her neurologist prescribed Tegretol, an additional anti-seizure medication. She did not suffer from delirium as during the onset of the previous seizures.

Remarkably, Maggie became hypo-manic a month after the third seizure and was seen on an emergency basis. Speaking rapidly, she was "grandiose," saying she wanted to drive alone to distant places, go shopping alone, and leave Richard because he was "too controlling." The doses of Tegretol and Haloperidol were increased, and the symptoms subsided within ten days. It remained unclear what caused these hypo-manic symptoms.

Maggie has continued to do well for the past six years. Her neurologist continues monitoring her anti-seizure medications on a regular basis. She is stable on twice daily doses of Tegretol 400 mg and Dilantin 200 mg. Two years after her last seizure, I substituted the Haloperidol with Risperdal 2 mg and kept the rest of her medications the same. The result was a lessening of her tiredness during the day. She takes Alprazolam only as needed. With a sharp mind, stable mood, and good memory, Maggie continues to read the newspaper, do crosswords puzzles, and more importantly, "enjoy life."

CHAPTER 16

High School Coach

The only completely consistent people are the dead.

Aldous Huxley

At six feet, ten inches tall, 210 pounds, blond and blue-eyed, Monty was a handsome, athletic 25-year-old young man when he first came into my office with his wife, Ginny. They had been married a little over a year.

It was the first time Monty had ever visited a psychiatrist. He said he was "stressed out." Ginny had been working away from home in Virginia Beach for the summer, and they were having marital conflicts. His parents were separating after being married for 35 years. Monty was working as a history teacher and head football coach in a high school that was in the midst of some racial tension. Like many young couples, their financial state was a primary stress: credit cards spent to their limit and unable to secure a loan for a new home, and they still wanted a new Corvette and better furniture.

Monty said he did not suffer from any physical problems, and denied abuse of alcohol or drugs, only drinking beer socially when he was watching ball games.

Monty's mother is a school teacher, and his father is a minister in a small church in Virginia. He sometimes drinks a lot and spends lot of money. Monty's older sister is a recovering alcoholic.

Monty has an undergraduate degree in coaching and history, as well as a graduate degree in counseling, both from the University of North Carolina.

I recommended first that he see a therapist in my office, individually and with his wife. Then, in less than three weeks, Monty became delusional that he was communicating with God. He wanted to get involved in politics, advocating freedom of choice, and wanted to go on national television. He thought that there was going to be a war between city boys and country boys, and he wanted to prevent it. He wasn't able to focus on any single thought. He was afraid of going to sleep. He was clearly manic, working for 16 to 18 hours at a time on several projects that he was not able to complete. He was very suspicious, and felt that people were following him. He started cutting out cartoons from the newspaper and writing illegibly.

He was voluntarily admitted to the hospital. He went through a thorough physical examination with complete labs and a urine drug screen, along with psychosocial and nursing assessment. His labs were normal; his drug screen was positive for marijuana.

Monty was initially treated with Haloperidol and Lorazepam to bring his manic and psychotic symptoms under control. He was given Restoril for sleep as needed. He was also started on Lithium Carbonate, and it was increased gradually from 600 mg to 1800 mg per day, while decreasing Haloperidol from 15 mg to 2 mg per day. He had no side effects from these changes. Several meetings were held with his wife to monitor his progress. Then, after eight days of being in the hospital, an overnight pass was given to see if his thinking and behavior were within the normal range of his natural environment. Ginny was pleased with his progress. Monty was discharged from the hospital the following day with Haloperidol 2 mg at night, and Lithium Carbonate 600 mg three times a day. His lithium blood level at the time of discharge was in the range of 0.81 meq per liter.

The final discharge diagnosis was Bipolar Affective (Manic Depressive) Disorder, manic phase.

A week later Monty came to see me with Ginny and stated that he was feeling "a thousand times better." He was thinking clearly and talking coherently. He had no grandiose schemes of rescuing the world, and he was not paranoid. He had gone back to work. He had no problems teaching. He denied abuse of alcohol or drugs. His Haloperidol was discontinued and we set an appointment for a month later.

Initially Monty had no side effects while taking 1800 mg per day of Lithium Carbonate; his lithium blood level was 0.90 meq per liter. He had gained 10 pounds. His sleep and appetite were normal, his teaching and coaching at school were going well, his mood and thoughts were improving, and he had no sexual side effects. Six weeks later, however, Monty complained of mild hand tremors and diarrhea. He was doing well at home, school, and in social settings. I recommended reducing the dose of Lithium

Carbonate gradually to 1200 mg per day, and told him to come see me in two to three months.

Monty continued to make satisfactory progress. His lithium blood level was at 0.6 meq per liter, and his thyroid profile was unchanged and within normal range. During the summer, he traveled to Las Vegas, California and Mexico. He also visited his sister in Arizona, who was under the care of a psychiatrist. His job and relationship were going well. His wife got another job, and they bought a house. I continued to see Monty at three- to four-month intervals.

Because he was doing so well, by 1995 we had reduced his Lithium Carbonate gradually, down to 600 mg per day. He continued to do well, and had no recurring symptoms of mania or depression. A year later, the Lithium Carbonate was further reduced to 300 mg per day. But within a week, Monty had trouble with his sleep, so he went back to 600 mg. He remained stable. His lithium blood level was 0.3 meq per liter.

Monty was getting tired of teaching and coaching. Finally, he quit school in August 1997, and started working at a distribution center and doing odd jobs. In view of his new stressors, I increased his dose of Lithium Carbonate to 900 mg per day. In December of that year, he started working for a national bakery, distributing bread all over the city from 4 A.M. in the morning until 2 P.M. It was a very physical work, and he liked it as there was more pay with all the benefits. I increased the Lithium Carbonate to 1200 mg per day again and started seeing him every month or two.

Monty remained stable, despite working very hard from 4 a.m. to 4 p.m. He had no recurrence of mania, delusions or depression. The following summer, he started to look for another job. He finally got a teaching post in a high school. He was happy and stable.

I had been discussing switching from Lithium to Depakote, and finally Monty was ready to transition during the summer of 1999. He tolerated the change well. He remained stable at Depakote 750 mg per day for six months. He was diagnosed with hiatus hernia and acid reflux. He was also more stressed at work. He wanted to go back on lithium, and thus was transitioned in January 2000. He remained stable at lithium carbonate 900 mg per day with a blood level of 0.5 meq per liter.

In fall of 2000, Monty started having marital problems. I recommended marital therapy to which he complied, but it did not work. He moved out of the house in May 2001. They were together for 13 years, and married for 10 years. I increased lithium carbonate to 1200 mg per day. He continued to remain stable.

With his good looks and stable job, Monty had no problems with dating, and engaging in sexual activity. He started drinking socially. Over holidays he felt lonely, and slightly depressed. His parents had been divorced for 10 years, and his father was getting married for the third time at the age of 65. He remained close to his mother, sister and a few friends. His divorce was final in January 2002.

Monty did well for about 11 years, until he stopped taking his medications properly, and began drinking and smoking marihuana more frequently.

During the summer he went on vacation with his girl friend, Monika, who is a social worker and 7 years younger than him. Monika liked alcohol and smoking pot. At her urgings, Monty became non compliant with lithium as his sex was slightly better without medications. He became more assertive and defiant in his behavior. I cautioned that he must reduce his drinking and abuse of marihuana, and go back on lithium; otherwise, he would end up in the hospital.

Within two days of Monty's visit to my office, I got a call from the Principal of his school that he was exhibiting bizarre behavior, and was not able to function. In view of this I immediately recommended hospitalization. He was taken by his father to a psychiatric hospital where he spent a week. He was stabilized on Depakote 2000 mg per day.

After his discharge from the hospital I continued to see Monty and monitor his medications. He has been functioning well at his work, and his relationship with Monika is going well. He drinks alcohol socially, and denies smoking marijuana. He has no sexual problems. He has been stable on Depakote 500 mg, and lithium carbonate 600 mg. He denies any side effects from the medications.

Monty wanted to be close to his mother. He successfully transitioned his job as a teacher. Monika wants to move with him, and they plan to live together. I have advised him to be compliant with medications, and be under the care of a psychiatrist who can monitor him on a regular basis.

CHAPTER 17

Psychotic Executive

On your journey, if you come upon a canyon in your path, jump. It is not as far as you think.

Native American Proverb

When I met Jody, she was a 38-year-old, slender, attractive divorced woman who worked in the accounting department of a reputable insurance company. She had been brought to the hospital in October 1997 by her supervisor, the manager of Human Resources, for odd behavior.

She said that her job had been becoming increasingly stressful. She traveled a lot, and had recently had to take time off because of stress. She said that odd things had been happening in her life for nearly two months. She believed that there was somebody beside her in the house, someone who was there to get her. She believed that someone was moving her things around. She noticed footprints outside the house. She also believed that at work, someone was changing the numbers on her computer. She felt like someone was trying to sabotage her work. She was getting calls from people she didn't know, and thought she was being followed by a black car. She didn't feel safe. She had called the police, who checked the house and found nothing out of the ordinary.

Jody was very paranoid, and did not want to talk about anything unless it was absolutely confidential. She had called her father, and he came from Georgia to be with her.

Jody said she'd never had any of these symptoms before. When I first saw her, she had minor depressive symptoms, namely problems with sleep, not eating as well, and feeling sad and fearful since onset of her paranoid and delusional symptoms. She was not having visual hallucinations or hearing voices. She said she didn't abuse alcohol, drugs, caffeine or cigarettes. She was not taking any prescribed or over-the-counter medications. She wasn't hearing any special messages from television or radio. She also denied any panic, obsessive-compulsive, or manic symptoms currently or in the past. She was alert and oriented to time, place and person. She was pleasant and cooperative. Her memory was intact, and her speech was linear and goal-oriented. Her mood was slightly sad under the circumstances, and she was quite guarded.

She was born and raised in Boston, Massachusetts. She has an MBA from Boston University. She was married for two years and has no children. She was not in a relationship at the time. She had moved to Charlotte five years earlier, and said her job was a good one. She had a good support system of friends, parents, family and coworkers and was very social. Her parents separated when she was 20 year old, but she says she had a very good childhood and there was no abuse of any kind. She has an older brother and an older sister. Except for her paternal grandfather drinking alcohol heavily, there was no history of alcohol, drug abuse or psychiatric illnesses in the family.

Jody had had some counseling in the past regarding relationship issues, but this was her first contact with a psychiatrist, and her first hospitalization. We did a thorough physical examination with complete analysis of blood and urine samples. Lipids, cholesterol, thyroid, and electrolytes were within normal range. All tests were negative, including the urine drug screen.

Based upon the clinical findings, a diagnosis of Paranoid Delusional Disorder, along with Major Depressive Disorder- mild, was given.

During this hospitalization, Jody received daily individual and group psychotherapy. She was started on a low dose of Haloperidol 1 mg orally at night, along with Trazodone 25 mg at night for sleep. We held a meeting with her father and mother when they came to visit her. The rationale for our diagnosis and prescription of medications was explained to them, and we discussed other concerns. Jody was started on a low dose of Prozac, 10 mg daily. Gradually her sleep, appetite, and mood started to improve, and her paranoid symptoms and fears started to subside. She felt confident, and had no thoughts of hurting herself or others. She was transitioned from Inpatient to the Day hospital after five days.

With the help of her family and friends, Jody continued to make steady progress. Her medications were continued and monitored for any side effects. She was able to sleep without

Trazodone, and it was discontinued. Further, she was able to discuss her stressors at work and in relationships in group therapy. She also learned a lot about her condition as well as other psychiatric conditions from the experiences of other patients. She learned how to cope and deal with her stressors. In view of the progress, she was discharged from the Day program after a week, and continued on Haloperidol I mg at night and 10 mg Prozac daily.

Within two weeks Jody came to see me in the office. She was elegantly dressed and groomed in professional attire. She was pleasant, smiling and cooperative. She was driving without any fear, and she had gone back to work part time. She had started to gain back her confidence at work and at home. She was sleeping and eating well. Her thinking was clear and sharp. She had no paranoid or delusional symptoms, and she was interacting well at work and in social settings. She had no side effects from the medications. She was seeing her therapist weekly.

At her next visit, after three weeks, Jody was making satisfactory progress. She had gone back to work full time. She was functioning at almost 100% of her capacity. She had no symptoms of depression or paranoia. Her dose of Haloperidol was reduced to 0.5 mg at night.

Jody continued to make progress, and I continued to see her once a month. She started dating, and she took a Dale Carnegie course to improve her business and human relations skills. She started to go to the gym and do regular exercise. She was traveling in her work without any problems. I discontinued her Prozac in March 1998, because of sexual side effects, and continued her on the Haloperidol 0.5 mg at night.

Jody began a relationship, and her boyfriend did not like her taking any medications. Based upon her history, it was not clear whether her psychiatric symptoms were only a one-time occurrence. Therefore, I decided to gradually reduce her Haloperidol to 0.25 mg for a month, and then allow her to go off of it.

Jody did well without any medications for three months. Her relationship was going well. She bought a townhouse. She got a promotion to manager of Customer Relations. She was happy and had no psychiatric symptoms.

Then, in 1998, she got a new supervisor with whom she had some conflict at work. She started to worry more, and her depressive symptoms started to creep in. She was concerned that her psychotic symptoms may come back. Thus she was started back on a low dose of Haloperidol and Prozac in August 1998.

The medications seemed to allow Jody to do better at work as well as in her relationship. But because of sexual side effects, she was taken off the Prozac in October 1998, and the Haloperidol was again gradually reduced to 0.25 mg.

Jody went through a phase of deterioration of the relationship with her boyfriend. He came from a different background and had fluctuating mood swings. Finally, she had the courage to break up without feeling guilty. During this phase, she continued psychotherapy and started back on a low dose of Prozac. It took her almost six months to get over this relationship.

In September 1999, she got a new job as vice president of Risk Management at a bank, and she started taking classes at Queens University in financial planning.

I discussed with Jody all along the atypical second generation antipsychotic medications, to get her to at least try one and see if it might suit her better. Although her dosages have been very small, she finally agreed in June 2000 to substitute Haloperidol with Risperdal at 0.25 mg. Initially she had difficulty in waking up in the morning, but she gradually got used to it. Overall, she feels less tired during the day on Risperdal.

Jody has been leading a successful and happy life since then. She has been traveling to foreign countries, dating, enjoying her friends and socializing, and doing very well in her job. I see her in my office once every two to three months. She is very stable on Prozac 10 mg and Risperdal 0.25 mg, without experiencing any side effects. She has good insight into her illness, and understands the role of medications in keeping her symptom-free and functioning optimally.

CHAPTER 18

An Actresses' Story

What I dream of is an art of balance.

Henry Matisee

When Heather first came to see me in April 2001, it was her first contact with a psychiatrist, though she had been in therapy for more than 22 years. My first impressions were that she was an attractive 48-year-old, well-nourished, single, African American female, five feet seven inches tall weighing 140 pounds, and dressed and groomed elegantly. She was referred by her therapist.

She described a life-long history of depression and anxiety. Her goal in therapy had been to separate herself from her mother; she had not been successful. For the past few years she had been in a group therapy as well. She said she was anxious all the time. She was a part-time stage performer, but felt anxious with people she does not know. She felt sad, hopeless, was tearful at times, had trouble concentrating and staying focused.

Heather was in menopause and was using progesterone cream. About 10 years earlier she had taken Prozac for a month and had lost 15 pounds and had problems sleeping. Paxil made her heart race and left her feeling hyper and even more anxious. On Klonopin, she was not able to get out of bed for a few days, and Pamelor also gave her severe side effects. Based upon these experiences, she was scared of medications. She had been drinking two glasses of wine every night for the past 18 years, smoked about four cigarettes per day but didn't do other drugs, including caffeine or over-the-counter medications.

As far as her history, Heather said she'd had no suicide attempts or suicidal thoughts, no obsessive-compulsive symptoms, paranoia, delusions or hallucinations. She had rheumatic fever as a child, but wasn't experiencing any physical problems, other than the menopause.

Heather's mother was 78 years old and suffered from anxiety. Her father died at 70. Her paternal grandfather was hospitalized for depression. One of Heather's two brothers was diagnosed with attention deficit disorder.

Heather was born in Gary, Indiana, moved to Baltimore, Maryland, and then to Washington, D.C. She was in Los Angeles for 15 years during her 20s and 30s, and then moved to Charlotte, NC. She has a bachelor's degree from the University of Maryland in Fine Arts. Heather had a good childhood, but says that her father physically abused her after they moved away from Gary. She also suffered emotional abuse from her family. There was one incident of sexual abuse by her older brother when she was 13.

She was working as an executive secretary with a national bank when she came to see me. She also worked as an actor in local theaters. She has never been married and has no children. She had two long-term relationships; one ended about three years before she came to my office. She described her stressors at the time as the anxiety and the depression. Her support system was limited to one friend and her therapist. Her strengths include being attractive, intelligent and having a good job.

I diagnosed her as having Generalized Anxiety Disorder and Major Depressive Disorder, with possible Alcohol Dependence of a mild form. I believed it was possible that she was drinking alcohol to alleviate her anxiety. She appeared to be very sensitive to the dosage of medications; therefore, after educating her about her diagnosis and the rationale for medication, I started her on Zoloft 25 mg per day and gave her a return appointment in two weeks.

Heather said the anxiety and depression had lessened by this second session. She was able to read a book. She was feeling hopeful. Her migraine headaches were better. Her sleep and appetite were not affected. She had no problem with her sexual desire , but had problems with getting orgasm. Her weight was unchanged. She had no other side effects. I continued Zoloft at the same dosage, and gave her an appointment in a month.

At this session Heather stated that for the past three weeks she had been experiencing nausea, diarrhea, cramps, and sleep problems. Her anxiety came back although she had reduced her drinking to an occasional single glass of wine. Her sexual problems had worsened. So I reduced her Zoloft to 12.5 mg and gave her a prescription of Alprazolam 0.25 mg to take one fourth to one half , as needed, for anxiety.

At the follow-up session in a month, Heather's mood, anxiety and functioning were better, and she said she had taken a fourth of the Alprazolam 0.25 mg four to five times the entire month. She had no side effects. She started to go back to group therapy sessions to work on her social anxiety. She was offered another job with more pay, and she was happy. I continued medications at the same dosages and gave her an appointment in two months.

Heather continued to make progress with her mother, and went to visit her after five years. She got a lead role in a play, and her new job was going well. She continued to make more friends, and became socially less anxious. She was also able to take more risks socially. She started going to more parties. She finally started to do Yoga and get regular exercise. She started to date again, and felt less anxious. She was able to withstand day-to-day stressors well. Because she was doing so well at such low dosages, she was tempted to go off the medications completely. She stopped taking them for about a month, and all her symptoms came back, so she quickly got back on them.

I continue to see her regularly once in two to three months.

There is a population of patients who are exquisitely sensitive to the regular dosages of medications as recommended by the FDA or manufacturers. These patients suffer because many physicians, instead of decreasing the dosages, tend to increase them so as to get better effectiveness, not realizing that the side effects especially of psychotropic medications become worse, with the result many patients stop taking them, and thus go on suffering. I have consciously picked up these cases in my stories so as to illustrate this point.

It is interesting, for example, that the manufacturer Eli Lilly of Prozac, one of the most successful antidepressant, when it came first on the market in 1989, had only one dose of 20 mg in capsule form so that one could not break it. Besides, being a good drug, 15 to 20% of the patients had severe side effects at 20 mg. It took 4 to 5 years for the manufacturer to come up with 10 mg tablets which could be broken into one half.

Likewise, when Risperdal came into the market, there were only 1 mg and 3 mg tablets. Much later the manufacturer Janssen realized the problem, and came up with lower dosages of 0.25 mg and 0.5 mg.

Another case in point is that a very useful medication, Klonopin, known for over 20 years has been dispensed as the smallest dose of 0.5 mg. For many patients even one half of this was too much. Only recently in 2003, a manufacturer came up with 0.25 mg.

In clinical trials, very sick patients from medical centers are enrolled, and they are excluded from testing if they have other accompanying psychiatric problems than the targeted one. Further, the dosage of medications needed to treat this population is generally higher than the patients treated in the office settings. In other words, medications for FDA purpose are tested with only one diagnosis generally with very sick patients. In real life, patients could have multiple diagnosis, such as substance abuse, panic disorders, OCD, depression, paranoia, explosive disorder, and premenstrual symptoms. In order for a patient to feel completely well, a physician thus has to make intelligent decisions not only with choices of medications, but also with their dosages.

CHAPTER 19

Am I Becoming Like My Mother?

Art is a revolt against fate.

Andre' Malraux

When Beth came to see me in January 2000, at the repeated urgings of her therapist, she was 40 years old. She was scared to see a psychiatrist. She had bad memories of her mother, who was agoraphobic and had panic attacks. Her mom had been committed to a state hospital when Beth was 3 years old and treated with electro-shock therapy.

For months, Beth had been feeling anxious and depressed, was irritable, crying a lot, felt scared. She wasn't functioning well at work or in social settings. She was afraid of elevators and heights. She was unable to drive long distances. She had been having panic attacks for 24 years, and depression for 20.

She was afraid she was turning into her mother.

When I diagnosed Beth with Panic Disorder with Agoraphobic features and Major Depressive Disorder, recurrent, she was afraid that she would ultimately get as bad as her mother. She was also afraid for her children's mental well-being.

Beth is a widow. She is scared of dating and has no current relationship. She lives with her children. She got married for the first time at age 26. She was married for eight years before her husband left her for another woman. She became a single mother with two small children, a mortgage, and a full-time job. She married for the second time at age 35. Her husband died of cancer two years later. Her father and stepfather are also dead.

Her father, who worked as an auto mechanic, used to drink heavily. He died at 65 of prostate cancer. Beth's mother suffered from agoraphobia and anxiety attacks; she also had bad tempers, and used to drink heavily. Beth is the only child. Her parents divorced when she was 12 years old.

Beth describes bad memories of her mother: "The earliest memory of my mother was of her jumping out of the car and running into the darkness. My father was petrified with fear, and he pleaded with her to get back into the car.

"My mother had me at age 18. When I was 3, she was committed to the state hospital, where she received electro-shock therapy. I was fearful as a child that I would be strapped down, have a rubber piece inserted into my mouth so as not to bite my tongue, and shocked to the point of losing my breath into unconsciousness.

"She suffered from panic attacks, and was afraid of open spaces. She would stay in her room for days. She became fearful of picking me up from school, going to the grocery store, or driving a car. She was explosive, screaming and yelling at the most trivial events. I thought that this was her release, a venting of anger, but it took a toll on everyone around her.

"When my parents divorced, my mother and I were left to take care of each other. I basically took care of both of us. She was a smart person trapped by her emotions and physiology. She could not drive into Charlotte and ride the elevators. As there was no proper medical help in the 1960s and 70s, she began to drink. This would alleviate some of the anxiety but added to the depression. In 1973, she tried to take her life by swallowing Librium and vodka. I called my aunt, who called the ambulance. She was taken to the hospital, where her stomach was pumped.

"In the meanwhile, the stress on a 14-year-old was taking its toll. I had continual stomach problems, and did not know at the time that I was suffering from a mild depression. I began to drink with my friends, smoke cigarettes, and went from an A student to a C and D student. I felt sorry for my mother and myself. I had no goals and no plans. I lived day by day."

Beth was a responsible and hard-working student. She was determined to fight her illness and her genetics. She read a lot of self-help books. She could not go to college as she had to go to work to support her mother. She began to work a night shift and attend a local college during the day. Finally she graduated at age 28 with a bachelor's degree in Biology. She worked for a utility company for 15 years, and now she works for the Department of Labor in human safety.

Beth drank alcohol heavily from age 20 to 25. She smoked a half a pack of cigarettes a day for 20 years but stopped about three months ago. Caffeinated drinks make her hyper. She has no medical problems and doesn't take over-the-counter medications. She is allergic to morphine.

In 1993, she was prescribed Zoloft, on which she had severe side effects. In 1997, she was given samples of Paxil; she experienced severe anxiety and panic attacks. And on Prozac, in 1999, she became paranoid and suicidal with anxiety attacks. Buspar gave her headaches. With these bad side effects, she has become fearful of medications. She is reluctant to try any new medications.

I educated Beth about her diagnosis and a possible genetic link to her parents' illnesses. She was shocked with my conclusion even though I was confirming what she had suspected all along. She asked me point blank: "Am I going to become like my mother?"

I wanted to be realistic but also empathetic. I told her that I am not sure. However, based on my experience of seeing thousands of patients and getting their family history, I am convinced that we not only inherit from our parents our external physical features but also internal biochemistry including the brain. And it is the brain chemistry that determines to a large extent who we are and how we deal with our stressors. This does not mean that the environment has no influence. On the contrary, the fine interplay between genetics and environment is crucial. Depending on what kind of supportive family, friends, school, community, culture, religion we have, as well as the coping mechanisms for stressors, the influence of genetics can be ameliorated.

Beth felt slightly better with my explanation. She was not fully satisfied. She has been a fighter, and she does not want this illness to be inherited by her children.

Based on her history she was exquisitely sensitive to medications and she must start with the lowest possible dose. I gave her a sample package of Remeron along with a prescription of Alprazolam 0.25 mg, a quarter to a half to be taken as needed for anxiety.

We scheduled a return appointment for 10 days, but Beth didn't show up for three weeks. She complained that she slept for two days on Remeron 7.5 mg, and then felt groggy the next day. However, she had started to eat better with no nauseous feeling. She stopped taking this medication and became scared of trying Alprazolam. She mentioned in passing that she had taken Tranxene 3.75 mg ½ to ¼ as needed about eight years ago, and had no problems. I immediately agreed and wrote a prescription. I educated her again on her diagnosis and the rationale of medications.

Beth did not return for her next appointment. She showed up nine months later, in November 2000. She wasn't taking any medications except small doses of Tranxene as needed. This was more helpful than Alprazolam.

Her anxiety was becoming unbearable as she was to go to a meeting for her job in Raleigh, N.C., about 180 miles away from her home. She was scared of driving that far. She had been listening to her meditation and agoraphobia tapes several times a day, but they were not helping. She was also stressed because her mother had been diagnosed with colon cancer and a surgery was scheduled. Her children and job were doing well. She was still not dating. She was fearful of getting emotionally involved. She also complained of premenstrual symptoms of easy tearfulness and some depression, lasing for four to five days.

I educated her again about the role of SRI medications and gave her a sample package of Paxil 10 mg, to take only a quarter before her menstrual cycle.

At her next session in a month, Beth stated that she had taken extra Tranxene before her PMS and it helped. She did not try Paxil due to her bad past experiences. She drove to Statesville, N.C. about 50 miles away, became anxious and came back. She was awfully anxious of traveling to Raleigh for the meeting. This time I gave her a prescription of Prozac 10 mg capsule to dissolve in orange juice. I told her to start with only 1 mg daily, and then increase to 2.5 mg after a week.

Beth was scared of trying Prozac. She increased her dose of Tranxene on her own, especially when she had to travel. She ventured up to 100 miles in different directions, such as Winston Salem, N.C., Greenville S.C., Salisbury N.C. successfully, but remained fearful of traveling up to Raleigh as she had a panic attack in that city.

Recently she had a panic attack in a dentist's office. She was happy otherwise. She had received a promotion at work. Her children were doing well in school. She still had no relationship, and was scared of dating.

She was encouraged to drive more to places where she had panic attacks so as to desensitize herself. I also recommended that she take Tranxene daily rather than as needed, and also to take an extra dose if she had to make a long trip. She was also cautioned to make sure that she was not feeling drowsy or sleepy, and that her alertness was not affected.

Beth continues to see me once every two or three months. She remains scared of trying SRI medications due to her past experiences. Sometimes, she takes her medication on a regular basis and then goes off for few weeks.

Overall she has done well. She has driven to Raleigh several times, and stayed in a motel, something that she had never done in the past. She also drove to Wilmington, N.C., 250 miles away to a conference from her work, and stayed there for five days. These are accomplishments that she is proud of. She is still not able to fly, go boating or go on a cruise.

Beth eventually started dating. She has been going out with a guy who is eight years younger. She is still scared of sexual involvement, as she had no sex in four years.

She has been happy at work. She has received another promotion. She is feeling more confident. I have been encouraging her to seek psychotherapy to get over the rest of her fears. She is reluctant and fearful to engage in psychotherapy, as she is fearful of trying different medications. She wants to do things in her own way, and I have no problem with that.

In one of the sessions, Beth told me that her 12-year-old son is showing signs of claustrophobia; she wonders whether he is going to have the same illness that she has. He had no physical or emotional traumas as compared to what she went through as a child. She has been a good provider. She did not bring any abusive boyfriends home. His father did not drink alcohol, and there is no history of depression, anxiety or panic attacks with him. So why should he get this illness?

From this story it is apparent that Beth is very scared of trying any new or old medications on which she had side effects. Despite my numerous reassurances she remained very reluctant to try. Further, she was able to adjust her medications according to her needs to which I had no objection as long as she was making progress.

Tranxene (Clorazepate) is in the benzodiazepine family of medications. Other members in the same family are Alprazolam (Xanax), Lorazepam (Ativan), Clonezapam (Klonopin), Diazepam (Valium), Oxazepam (Serax), Chlordiazepoxide (Librium), Temazepam (Restoril), etc. These medications are very useful in the management of anxiety, panic and sleep disorders.

This story further illustrates the uniqueness of individual biology, and how people respond differently to medications.

CHAPTER 20

Obsessed With Changing Clothes, And Making Detailed Notes

And I show you something different from either
Your shadow at morning striding behind you
Or your shadow at evening rising to meet you;
I will show you fear in a handful of dust.

T. S. Eliot

Virginia, a 52-year old attractive Hispanic, who goes by the name Ginny, had been in therapy for 31 years before she had any contact with a psychiatrist. She slit her wrists at the age of 19 when she was in college, and was sent to see a psychologist. She went to her first therapist when she was 21. She had a history of being shy and nervous her whole life, of having headaches and suicidal thoughts. She had never been hospitalized. She had been treated for years for depression and anxiety by her primary care doctors.

Ginny was referred to my office in January 2002. She'd begun seeing her current therapist a decade earlier, when she was diagnosed with breast cancer and underwent a lumpectomy and radiation therapy. Physically, she was healthy when she first came to see me. But she said her overall functioning was about in the middle on a scale from 1 to 10. She was very sad about having suffered for so long despite therapy and medications. On the same scale, 10 having no psychiatric symptoms, and 1 being the worst, she rated herself around "8" for depression, about a "5" for paranoia and "odd feelings," between "2 to 3" for anxiety and obsessive-compulsiveness.

Ginny told me at that initial visit that she'd been obsessed about changing her clothes several times a day for years -- even in college. She also makes very detailed notes about everything since high school; she has volumes of notes at home. For most of her life, she believed someone was watching her. She has been very self-conscious of feeling different, thinking different, and being "unique" from others. In high school, she was anorexic. She has been nervous all her life. She is afraid of crowds, people, and being trapped in elevators. She denied having experienced a panic attack or manic symptoms. She smoked marijuana in high school and college and it helped her symptoms. She drinks alcohol socially but doesn't smoke cigarettes, or use any recreational drugs.

I diagnosed Ginny with Major Depressive Disorder with possible mild psychotic features, Generalized Anxiety Disorder, and Obsessive Compulsive Disorder. Once we worked out the proper combination and dosages of medicines, she began to feel less anxious, calmer, more organized and less distracted than ever before. She was confident and less fearful. She stopped writing so many detailed notes and changing her clothes so often.

Ginny is the only child in her family. Physically she is like her mother – slender, beautiful -- but emotionally, she is like her father. He suffered from very bad anxiety and depression and attempted suicide a few times. His own mother suffered from depression and was treated with electroshock therapy. Both parents are 73 years old. They are retired and live in Georgia.

Ginny was born in El Paso, Texas and raised in Georgia. She moved all over the country growing up. She describes her childhood as good, although her parents were very strict. There was some emotional abuse by her parents, but no physical or sexual abuse.

She has a bachelor's degree in general education. She married at the age of 23. Her husband is 54 years old and works as an accountant for local bank. Her 21-year-old son suffers from depression as well. Ginny worked in a local hospital, and at the beginning of our sessions, she was working part time. She has a good support from her husband and church. Her major stress was the illness of her father.

In 1988, Ginny was treated by her primary care physician for depression with Imipramine, and she did well. In 1994, she was treated with Buspar for anxiety. In 1996, she had a severe reaction from one dose of Paxil 20 mg -- she passed out, had seizure-like activity, and started throwing up. In 1999, she was prescribed Effexor by her PCP. She continued to have side effects such as feeling nervous, having difficulty driving, and having minor car accidents. At higher dose of Effexor, Ginny began to feel lethargic along with other side effects.

At our first session, I reduced her dose of Effexor and gave her a prescription of alprazolam 0.25 mg as needed. A return appointment was given in two weeks. Ginny was less anxious and calmer while taking a lower dose of Effexor along with Xanax 0.25 mg one half in the morning and one in the evening. Her depression, focus, and concentration were better. She felt more confident with her driving. There was no change in her paranoia, so I gave her samples of Risperdal with a return appointment in two weeks.

Ginny said the 0.5 mg of Risperdal made her body slightly stiff, and she had difficulty walking, so she reduced it to 0.25 mg. She was calmer, less anxious, less distracted and more organized. Her paranoia was improving. She was less fearful and less self-conscious. She wrote fewer detailed notes, didn't change her clothes as much, and began to drive better. She said her husband, mother and pastor were noticing the difference in her behavior and attitude.

At her next visit in three weeks, Ginny continued to make progress. She was also seeing her therapist once a week. She went on vacation with her husband and did well. She denied any sexual problems. Her job was better. She was "rediscovering" herself, and getting a new life. Her primary care physician was happy that she was doing better.

I continued to see Ginny once a month. We adjusted Effexor XR to 150 mg when she became slightly depressed, and she continued to take the same amounts of Risperdal and Xanax.

Her symptoms of depression, paranoia, anxiety and obsessive-compulsive behavior continued to improve further. She was getting more confident, and started looking for a job with more responsibilities. Her hot flashes also started to improve. She accepted deacon's responsibilities at her church, and started teaching Bible classes.

During the course of her treatment she complained of low libido, possibly due to menopause. We tried a low dose of Wellbutrin, but even with half of what was prescribed, she became nervous and shaky and started to hallucinate, so it was stopped.

Ginny had a good Christmas and New Year. In January 2003, her mother had a stroke, and she went to Georgia to take care of her and her father who has dementia. She started moving back and forth between Charlotte and Georgia to take care of them. She took the responsibility of having power of attorney over their affairs. Her father was hospitalized several times. She was successful in relocating them to Charlotte and finding a nursing home for them. She is convinced that without the help of the proper medications, she would not have been able to handle the family stresses as well as she did.

Primary care physicians, internists, pediatricians and Ob/Gyn prescribe 70% of psychotropic medications for treatment of psychiatric disorders. They do a very good job for uncomplicated patients. For patients who have substance abuse, or have multiple psychiatric disorders, and are not getting well, a consultation with a psychiatrist can save years of trying different medications or prolonging their symptoms. Ginny is a good example of not having had the quality of life for decades, prior to her seeking proper help.

I very often hear from my physician colleagues that patients are afraid to seek help from psychiatrists, not only because of stigma, but also that their insurance premium would go up or they may not be able to get life or other insurances. This is a shame that the insurance companies think that patients who seek help from psychiatrists have a higher incident of committing suicide, and thus they are a high risk population. On the contrary, by seeking help from therapists and psychiatrists, patients have become more productive at work, at home and in social settings.

CHAPTER 21

I Have ADD!

Bear near me when the sensuous frame
Is raked with pains that conquer trust;
Tennyson

After a series of written tests, Paula's psychologist diagnosed her with Attention Deficit Disorder (ADD) in December 2002 and referred her to my office so that I would prescribe the "appropriate" medication. (Psychologists have no medical training to prescribe drugs.)

She assumed that I would simply prescribe the medication for ADD and that would be it. My diagnosis was different.

Paula is an attractive redhead in her early 50s. She had lost 7 pounds over the past two weeks. She is a professor of History at the local university. She has been in Charlotte for 20 years. She has been divorced for a year after 18 years of marriage to her husband, who teaches Art. They have two children, ages 10 and 14. They are going through a tough custody battle. She moved out of the house 18 months ago because of serious relationship problems. Her children stayed with their father.

She's confused. She does not remember names of friends and colleagues. She has been forgetting her appointments, despite making notes in her PDA. She wants to sleep a lot, and remains sleepy and inattentive during the day. She feels tired, withdrawn and is not functioning well at home or in school. She has taken a semester off from work so as to sort through her family and mental problems. She has lost 13 pounds in less than six months. She is still very depressed. Last year she was feeling suicidal.

A remarkable and noteworthy feature of her presentation, besides being very nervous and agitated, was her strange continuous staring into my face without blinking her eyes. Her personality and conversational style were very sticky. She had great difficulty in shifting to a different topic and letting go of things. She was quite confused and repeated herself frequently.

About 10 years ago, Paula was treated with Wellbutrin for two to three years. About 5 years ago she was treated with Prozac for a year. Since her separation, her primary care physician has given her Remeron and Ambien for sleep.

She has never been treated by a psychiatrist prior to this visit.

Paula said she doesn't feel suicidal or homicidal, wasn't obsessive compulsive and wasn't abusing drugs, cigarettes or alcohol. She denied any history of eating disorder or bad tempers and says she has no paranoia, hallucination or delusions.

On a scale of 1 to 10, 10 being the best and 1 being the worst, Paula described her functioning at work around 6, and at home and social settings around 4 to 5. On the same scale 10 being no depression, and 1 being worst, she rated herself around 3, and for general confusion around 3, as well.

Paula was born and raised in the Midwest. Her childhood was excellent. There was no physical, emotional or sexual abuse while growing up. Her parents are in their seventies, and they had their own real estate company. They are financially well off. Except for her younger sister, who suffers from depression, there is no history of depression or alcohol abuse in the family.

She has a master's degree in American History from the University of Minnesota. She got married at the age of 33. She has been extremely stressed over the legal battle regarding custody of her children. She is socially popular and has a good number of dependable friends.

I explained my diagnostic impression of severe Major Depressive Disorder. I also explained my rationale of selection of medications and their possible side effects. I took her off of Remeron, started her on Wellbutrin and continued Ambien for sleep as needed. A return appointment in two weeks was given.

Paula was still very depressed and confused. Her thought pattern was bizarre and illogical. She was not able to think clearly. Her thinking was slow, and her responses to my questions were also unusually slow. She was, however, alert and oriented to time, place and person. She continued to stare intensely at me.

These findings alerted me that her depression has psychotic symptoms. And she would not get well unless I treated her with an antipsychotic medication.

I explained my rationale of starting her on a low dose of Risperdal. She was very adamant that she has ADD, and became angry I was not treating her for that.

I explained to her again the hierarchy of most common psychiatric disorders: at the top level are medical and neurological illnesses, followed by alcohol and substance abuse, dementia, schizophrenia, bipolar affective disorder, clinical depression, obsessive compulsive disorder, anxiety and panic disorder, attention deficit disorder and personality disorders. She listened attentively but was not convinced. She told me again that her psychologist, with lot of paper and pencil tests, had determined that she had ADD, and thus she must be treated for that.

I gave her samples of Risperdal 0.5 mg to be added to the other medications. We made an appointment for her to return in two weeks. She called within two days requesting to be seen earlier. She had asked a pharmacist friend about Risperdal, who told her that it was for schizophrenia. Paula questioned my diagnosis, and asked why I was giving her this medication as she was not schizophrenic. She had gone to the Internet and made a copy of the diagnostic criteria of schizophrenia.

I explained again my rationale and experience in treating patients with these medications. Further I explained to her that the pharmacist and the psychologist are not psychiatrists, and they have no clinical experience in treating psychiatric disorders with medications.

Paula told me that her psychologist works with several primary care doctors, and makes recommendations for psychiatric medications to which they gladly comply. She said that if I was not going to treat her for ADD, she would go to the doctor that psychologist recommended, or she would find another psychiatrist. I was not surprised.

I know almost all the psychologists and therapists in the city. A good number of them do not refer patients to psychiatrists. They deal only with primary care doctors, and recommend them psychiatric medications. Further, they have been advised by their American Psychological Association to have a working relationship with the primary care doctors. And the APA has been trying to get prescription privileges for psychologists, not through medical training but through the legislative process of influencing the state legislatures.

The practice of psychiatry is both an art and a science. Besides a good basic knowledge of general medicine, it needs a strong knowledge of chemistry, biochemistry, physiology, pharmacology, brain anatomy and its chemistry, genetics, nutrition, neurology, and general theory and practice of contemporary psychiatry. Further, a physician must know the relation of psychiatry with other medical specialties, such as neurology, oncology, cardiology, gastroenterology, rheumatology, endocrinology and infectious diseases, just to mention a few. A psychiatrist spends four to five years of residency training to treat patients with acute and severe psychiatric disorders both in the hospital and outpatient settings. It is very unfortunate that our legislatures and lay public have no idea of the difference between a psychiatrist and psychologist. It is my personal belief that psychologists do not know and are not trained in even 25% of what I have mentioned above.

A clinical psychologist that I know tells people that the difference between a psychiatrist and psychologist is $40 an hour. It is a shame that the medical training and education of psychiatrists are undermined by psychologists, and their APA organization.

Paula listened very intensely and became convinced by my arguments; she agreed to take the Risperdal.

Before her next session in two weeks, she called me three times with trivial questions about medications. I was patient in answering her questions.

When we next met, Paula was calm and smiling. She did not stare at me as intensely. She had gone back to school and taught some classes. This was a major accomplishment as she had not taught in several months. She was able to concentrate and focus better. She had more energy and was sleeping better. Her mood was improving.

She was taking Wellbutrin 300 mg, Risperdal 0.5 mg and Ambien 10 mg. She complained of dry mouth as a side effect. She was pleased with the progress. But she was still reluctant to take anti-psychotic medication. I again educated her about the psychiatric illness and medications. She was more accepting as she was seeing the improvement. She continued to see her therapist with her children.

At the next session in two weeks, Paula brought her 72-year-old mother who was visiting from the Midwest. Paula was taking Wellbutrin 300 mg but only 0.25 mg of the Risperdal. She had reduced the dose to cut costs, although I had tried to help her with samples. I again summarized my findings from the chart to her mother, who pointed out that Paula was not sleeping well, was obsessing a lot, and got stuck with her thoughts easily and couldn't get away from them. She had done better on Prozac in the past. So I took her off of Wellbutrin, and started her on Remeron and Prozac, and continued on Risperdal.

Paula cancelled the next appointment and came after a month. She was elegantly dressed with appropriate makeup. She was driving without any problems. She had also started dating a guy who is eight years younger than her. She was functioning up to 80% of her capacity. She was teaching full time. She was able to plan her lessons well without getting confused. She was better able to plan her day without being late to appointments. She was gaining more self-confidence. She was not as obsessive. She was sleeping and eating better. She gained about 7 pounds in a month. I substituted Remeron with Trazodone to be taken as needed for sleep.

I continued to see Paula once a month for couple of months, and then once in two months. She continued to make improvements in her psychiatric symptoms, and thus in her work, and her relationship with her family and boyfriend. She started to look for other work which could bring more money. She also started to take advanced computer classes, and did well. She had no sexual side effects on Prozac 20 mg and Risperdal 0.25 mg. She again wanted to stop Risperdal because of its expense as it is not generic. I again cautioned her not to go off of it, and substituted it with Haloperidol. She liked this medication because of its low cost and the fact that for her, it had the same benefits.

It is not always possible to come to the right psychiatric diagnosis at the first session. As I get more information during the course of treatment, from the patient or other sources, I try to confirm, modify or change my diagnosis, and thus the treatment plan. In Paula's case, she not only suffered from depression but also had paranoia along with obsessive quality to her thinking. She does not have ADD, as determined by the psychologist with paper pencil tests. Therefore, every clinician must be very careful in the diagnosis as well as treatment choices.

CHAPTER 22

Praying 400 Times A Day

Your children are not your children.
They are the sons and daughters of Life's longing for itself.

Khalil Gibran

Frankie's father has been under my care since October 2000. He has been suffering from obsessive compulsive disorder along with depression and panic attacks. In the due course of his treatment, he mentioned that his 10-year-old son may have obsessive compulsive disorder as well. Normally I do not see children. But if I am treating either of the parents, I will make an exception.

Frankie was accompanied by his parents. He is in the fifth-grade at a public middle school. He is a very good student, and makes all A's. He has lots of friends and a best friend, Jonathan. He plays tennis and basketball. He gets along well with other students. He is very articulate and very intelligent.

His parents told me that for the past year, Frankie had been washing his hands excessively, at least 20 times a day. He repeats certain words several times. He prays a lot, sometimes up to 400 times a day. He is afraid of pictures on the wall, especially if they have black and red colors. He thinks these are evil colors. As a consequence of his obsessions and compulsions, he feels sad and has difficulty falling asleep. It is interesting to note that Frankie's father had similar symptoms as a child.

There is no abuse of cigarettes, alcohol or drugs by Frankie or his parents. Physically, Frankie is healthy and at 4 feet 10 inches, weighs 90 pounds. He does not take any medications.

His parents are well off, and they are college educated. His parents are undergoing some personal and professional stresses. Frankie has had a very good childhood. He is the only child. His father is a hospital administrator, and his mother is a school teacher. His grandparents live in Maryland, and they are also well off. He spends summers with his grandparents. There is no history of current or past trauma, or hardships.

In view of this history, I diagnosed Frankie with Obsessive Compulsive Disorder. I discussed the pros and cons of medication with him and his parents. They agreed to have at least a trial of a low dose of medication. Frankie's father had responded well to Prozac, so a low dose of 5 mg a day was started.

The dose of Prozac was gradually increased to 20 mg. Frankie's praying started to decrease from 400 times a day to 50 times per day. Further these prayers were of a much shorter duration. It was easier for him to say goodbye in the morning before going to school. He was not getting upset about not believing enough in God. His mood was better and his sleep and appetite were not affected. Overall he was happier.

Frankie also continued to see a therapist for dealing with the conflicts at home with his parents.

When Frankie reached puberty, his dose of Prozac was increased to 30 mg a day. He tolerated this without any side effects. He continues to make satisfactory progress.

There is a controversy all over the world about medicating children with powerful drugs to control their behavior or enhance their functioning. For parents, it is a huge question. There are pressures from school counselors, especially when a child is disruptive in class and defies rules at school or home, to seek help from professionals. The older generation wonders what is to become of a society when children are being medicated for long-term chronic illnesses such as depression, ADD/ADHD, bipolar, OCD, conduct disorder or substance abuse.

Genetically these disorders have been with us for thousands of years. Are there any biological advantages in the propagation of these disorders? How did previous generations cope with these conditions?

Besides genetics, what is the role of environment and lifestyle in the expression of these disorders at such an early age? Further, what roles are the media and the powerful pharmaceutical industry, along with physicians, playing in propagating the myth of a perfect and most intelligent child?

Scientists and clinicians are quite disturbed about these developments, and there are no easy answers.

There is no doubt that we have learned more about brain functioning and its chemistry during the past twenty years than during the rest of mankind's history. This knowledge – like the Human Genome Project -- has very serious implications for mankind. We could use this knowledge eventually to produce the most loving and intelligent human beings, but we could also use it to produce the most cruel and ruthless dictators.

It will thus be quite a challenge for this and the next generation, to regulate advances in brain chemistry to the benefit of mankind.

CHAPTER 23

First Pregnancy

An artist is a dreamer consenting to dream of the actual world.

George Santayana

Connie came to see me in March 2002 because she was paranoid, depressed and had no energy. The 33-year-old was referred through her insurance company.

In January 2001, Connie had started to hear voices, feel paranoid and depressed. She was treated in an outpatient setting with Risperdal and Celexa. She had taken the Celexa once before, for four years, because of depression and marital problems. By the time she came to see me, she was taking 40 mg of Celexa a day and 0.5 mg of Risperdal in the morning and 1 mg at night. She was sleeping 14 hours a day and had no sexual desire, no vaginal lubrication, and no orgasm. Further, her prolactin level was elevated, although her MRI scan of the brain was unremarkable.

Connie was well-nourished and physically healthy. She said she had never felt suicidal or obsessive-compulsive. She'd never been admitted to a psychiatric hospital. She had experienced no mania, no bad tempers. She wasn't using or abusing alcohol, marijuana, cigarettes, or excessive caffeine. She said that her overall functioning was good, a "7" on a scale of 1-10. But she was hearing voices, was paranoid and depressed. She was experiencing marital and sexual problems. Celexa had improved premenstrual symptoms, but left her with a host of other side effects, primarily the sexual problems.

Connie was adopted as a baby. She does not know her biological parents. Her adoptive parents are very well off, and they are in their early 70s. They do not drink or use drugs. They are very religious.

Connie was born in Omaha, Nebraska, and raised there. She had a wonderful childhood. She traveled with her parents to Europe and all over the United States. There was no physical, emotional or sexual abuse. Her parents moved to California when she was 10 year old. She had lots of friends in high school. She finished her undergraduate degree in psychology from UCLA. She got married at the age of 25, to her present husband, Mark, who is 33 years old. They have no children. Mark works for one of her father's software development companies. They relocated to Charlotte in August 2001. She works for her husband.

I diagnosed her with Major Depressive Disorder with Psychotic Features and reduced the amount of Risperdal she was taking. I explained my rationale for the reduction due to excessive sedation to 1 mg at night, and continued with the same dose of Celexa.

Three weeks later, Connie stated that she was not sleeping as much, and she had more energy. She was exercising more. She had lost four pounds. She was more alert and getting along better with Mark and other employees. Her mood was unchanged, and she had no psychotic symptoms. Despite these improvements, there was no change in her sexual dysfunction. I reduced the Risperdal further to 0.5 mg.

Connie lost another three pounds in three weeks. Her depression and psychotic symptoms were under control. There was no drowsiness during the day. She was exercising regularly, and getting along well with Mark. At this session I decreased her Celexa to 20 mg.

When I next saw Connie in a month, she was very happy. She had gone with Mark to Las Vegas and Los Angeles on a business trip. She enjoyed herself for the first time in a long time. She was free of all side effects. She wasn't sleeping as much, there were no hallucinations, delusions or paranoid feelings, and there was no milky discharge from her breasts, which had been plaguing her all along. She said she felt "free" as a woman. Now she was thinking of going off of birth control pills to get pregnant. She had lost four more pounds, and now weighed 134. I discussed medications and pregnancy and recommended that she come see me early if she got pregnant.

Two months later, Connie had gone back to full-time graduate school and was working part time. She said that about three weeks earlier, she had started experiencing some depression and hearing voices again. She was still taking the 20 mg of Celexa and 0.5 mg of Risperdal, but she had stopped taking birth control pills and had started to menstruate. She stated that when her prolactin level was high, she had stopped menstruating.

I increased her Celexa to 40 mg, and requested a blood prolactin level.

At Risperdal 0.5 mg, Connie's prolactin level was high -- 26.3 ng/ml. The normal range is 3 to 20 ng/ml. Her mood and psychotic symptoms were under control, she was getting along well with her husband and at her work, and she was happy with her studies. But because she was so sensitive to the Risperdal, we agreed to transition to another second generation antipsychotic drug to see how she would respond. I chose Seroquel.

Within the next few months, I increased Seroquel doses gradually up to 500 mg. Her symptoms had come back. She was mildly paranoid, had delusions of Mark having affairs, and was hearing the voice of God. She went to visit her parents over Christmas and missed taking her medications. She didn't sleep well, and became psychotic. She was stressed over school assignments as well. When she came home on New Year's Eve, she had to be taken to the Emergency Room because of increased psychotic symptoms. She was started back on Risperdal 1 mg and continued on Celexa.

Her psychotic symptoms came under control, but her blood prolactin level shot up to 66.7 ng/ml, and she stopped menstruating. On Seroquel 500 mg per day, she was having no problems with menstruation, but her psychotic symptoms resurfaced.

Connie stopped going to school as it was too stressful and went back to working full time. I reduced the Risperdal to 0.5 mg again and started her gradually on another second generation antipsychotic medication, Geodone increasing it gradually from 20 to 40 mg. Connie responded satisfactorily to the new medication. She had no paranoia, delusions or hallucinations, she had no discharge from her breasts, her menstruation resumed normally, her mood was better, and she had no sexual side effects. She was getting along well with Mark and her coworkers.

There was a concern about cardiac arrhythmia while on Geodone, so we performed an EKG. It was unremarkable.

I took Connie off the Risperdal and increased the dose of Geodone to 80 mg. She continued to do well without any side effects. Her weight was 136 pounds. She was exercising regularly. She went back to school.

I got a call from Connie in May 2003 that she was pregnant. I asked her to reduce the dose of Geodone gradually from 80 mg to 40 mg, and come to see me.

At her next session, Connie had been pregnant for three months. She was taking Celexa 40 mg and the Geodone. Her OB/GYN was aware of the medications and knew that he could call me any time. Connie had no symptoms of depression or paranoia. Her sleep was better, and she had no side effects.

Connie continued to see me once a month. She was due in January 2004. Her ultrasound test at five months of pregnancy was unremarkable; the baby was a girl. All other tests, such as that for Down syndrome, were negative. Her mood was better. She was doing water aerobics and exercising regularly. She was getting along with Mark. They were looking forward to a new life.

In September she came for her last visit. As her parents were getting old, and they had lot of property and business in California, Connie and Mark had decided to relocate. Connie was very happy with the decision as she wanted to be close to her parents. I recommended that she find a good psychiatrist, gave her a copy of my notes and wished her all the best.

CHAPTER 24

Indecent Exposure

Sex is something I really don't understand, too hot

. . . .

I keep making up these rules for myself, and then I break them right away.

J. D. Sallinger

Richard, who goes by the nickname "Dick," has had a lifelong obsession with public masturbation and pornography. He has been exposing himself in public since he was a teenager. He found me in the Yellow Pages a week after he was charged with indecent exposure in Virginia.

He had been charged with a similar offense when he was 18. He sought some therapy at that time, and again at age 25, when he had six months of psychotherapy with a psychiatrist. It was not very effective, and he went back to his same habits of not being able to control his sexual urges to expose himself and to engage in masturbation in public.

Dick is a 41-year-old, attractive, slender man. He's been married for 21 years; his wife Jean is very supportive.

The most recent charge stems from a business trip to Virginia. He was wandering in his truck early one evening when a police officer spotted him in a busy public area and caught him red-handed. He was arrested and spent the night in jail. He was released on bail and told to appear in court in a month.

When Dick came to see me he was depressed, guilty and sad, and was having some suicidal thoughts. He was sleeping and eating fine, and denied any plans to hurt himself. He doesn't have a bad temper, has had no paranoia, delusions or hallucinations. He denied any previous history of depression.

Jean knows about this incident.

Dick and Jean make love two to three times a week. He says he has never experienced sexual misconduct with minors, has no homosexual tendencies and does not have sex with prostitutes.

He's been smoking two packs of cigarettes per day for over 20 years. He drinks alcohol socially, smokes pot occasionally and denies abuse of other drugs. He had a physical examination recently, and his labs were normal. Further, he denied any concerns for HIV infection.

Dick was born and raised in Charlotte, N.C. He graduated high school and got married at the age of 20 to Jean. They have an 8-year-old son. He has been happy in the marriage. His wife works in the business that they own with three employees. He travels a lot in his business.

He is a good Christian, and the family belongs to a church.

His major stress has been the recent event in Virginia and his arrest. He has good support from his wife and family.

Based upon this information, I formally diagnosed him with Obsessive Compulsive Disorder, Adjustment Disorder with

Depressed Mood, and Nicotine Dependence. I started him on Paxil CR. I also strongly recommended psychotherapy.

At the return session two weeks later, Dick reported that he was not buying pornographic magazines, had not been riding around looking for women, and had not masturbated in public. Further, his mood was better, and he had no suicidal thoughts. He had no problems with desire for sex or achieving an erection; however, his orgasm was prolonged. His functioning at work, family or social life was not affected. I gave him a note that he has been under my care for his court hearing. He was continued on Paxil CR 25 mg. A return appointment was given in three weeks.

Dick continued to make satisfactory progress. He was more focused at work. His temper and mood were better. He had no incidents of exposing himself. His problems with orgasm continued. He started to smoke more than the two packs of cigarettes per day. I gave him a prescription for Wellbutrin to reduce his smoking and to help with sexual side effects.

Dick continued to improve, and I continued to see him every two or three months. His case was finally heard in court after a year. He had to pay a fine of $600 plus a lawyer's fee of $700. He stopped taking Wellbutrin and continued on Paxil CR 12.5 mg. He has been free of initial symptoms. He feels happy and amazed that one little pill could take away his life-long obsession with pornography and masturbation in public.

Medications belonging to Serotonin Reuptake Inhibitors, SRI (Prozac, Paxil, Zoloft, Celexa, Lexapro, Luvox) have been very useful in not only treating depression, but general and social anxiety, panic disorder, obsessive compulsive disorder, bulimia, premenstrual symptoms and premature ejaculation. The doses of SRI for treatment of these disorders are different, and they need to be individualized so as to minimize the side effects. Further, SRI could have serious side effects, and thus must be monitored carefully.

CHAPTER 25

Held By A Master: An Unfinished Story

And painful pleasure turns to pleasing pain.

Edmund Spencer

Tom had been going to bars all his adult life, alone or with friends. This time it was different. It was a nice summer evening. His girlfriend was working late, and he got finished early. Lately, he had been feeling a little down with the usual worries of money, work and relationships. He decided to go to a bar in a five-star hotel downtown. It was a little early for the bank people to crowd in. He was not a stranger to this place. He sat at the bar in a corner and ordered a whiskey with soda.

He noticed a tall, well-built, dark-skinned man watching him with steely eyes at the other end of the bar. He ordered another drink and got absorbed into his problems; his head was hanging down. Suddenly he noticed this man sitting next to him. The man introduced himself as Mustafa. He said he was a wealthy businessman from the Middle East who came to the city frequently. He owned an export-import business of sophisticated computers and had branches in London and Frankfurt. Tom was impressed. He had not met a person of such a standing in his life. He wished that Mustafa could become friends with him, thinking that may be one day he'd be able to see the world outside the United States.

Tom shared his life experience with Mustafa. He described being raised on a farm in South Carolina with his two sisters and told how, when he was 4 years old, his father was killed in a farming accident. His mother remarried when he was 8, and the family moved to Charlotte. His stepfather is a Presbyterian minister and was a very strict disciplinarian. Tom went to a community college and took courses in business. He was working as a manager of a fast food store. He wasn't married, and had no children. He lived with his girlfriend, who works for a bank. He found Mustafa to be a sympathetic listener, and caring.

Mustafa offered Tom another round of drinks; before they were finished he invited him to his suite. In his semi-drunken state, Tom accepted the invitation and followed him to his room.

The suite was spacious. It had its own bar, and an office area separate from the bedroom. Its windows opened into the skyline of the city, and Tom could see the sprawling new suburban developments. Mustafa ordered food from room service, along with a couple of bottles of French wine. Tom was impressed with his commanding style.

Tom had started drinking at the age of 13. He drank heavily from the age of 25 -- one, two or three bottles of wine a day. He had developed a high tolerance for alcohol.

After a light supper, Mustafa excused himself and took a quick shower. When he came out of the bathroom, he had no clothes except a long, thick white cotton robe. He smelled of musk perfume all over his body. Tom was relaxing on the sofa and enjoying his glass of wine. Mustafa toasted their new friendship. He was quite relaxed, and refilled the glasses with wine.

Then he came close to Tom, and started gently stroking his hair and face. Tom liked the attention and did not resist the advances. Mustafa gradually and deliberately untied his robe. Tom could not resist, and started playing with his hands and finally engaged in oral sex. In his 40 years he had never had such an experience. Mustafa told him to go to the bathroom and take a shower.

In the middle of the shower, Mustafa came into the bathroom, and they showered together, soaping each other and having another round of sex, this time anal. Again this was Tom's first experience, and he liked it.

They drank more wine. At that time Mustafa told Tom that he would be his "Master," that he would have full control of him. Tom must not tell anyone, not even his girlfriend, of their relationship without his permission. He would teach him more of the Eastern ways of how to be a man. He would take care of Tom.

They lay in bed for another couple of hours, until it was midnight. "Master" called the concierge for a cab for Tom to be taken home.

At the command of his Master, Tom went to different hotels on weekends. He was introduced to other Middle Eastern men who called Mustafa the Master and obeyed him. They had parties of drinking and sex. Most of the time, Tom was a receiver in sexual acts and quite passive.

These parties continued for a couple of months. Then Tom started feeling depressed and did not want to participate. At that time he told Master, who promised to look for a psychiatrist who understood their situation.

In the Yellow Pages, among the psychiatrists, my name is the most Eastern and exotic. Thus I was chosen by the Master for an appointment for Tom.

Tom is a 5-foot-7, chubby-looking white male who appeared younger than his age of 40. He weighed 157 pounds. He described the circumstances of his relationship with the Master and his friends in detail. He felt totally controlled by Mustafa. He was quite subdued. He did not want anyone to know of this special relationship. Neither his girlfriend nor any of his family or friends knew. He felt safe in the relationship. He did not feel any threat of harm to himself or others.

Tom then described a history of depression that had been going on for at least 25 years. He was depressed even in high school. Both his sisters are depressed, as well as the grandparents on his father's side. He self-medicated with alcohol but had never been treated with psychotherapy or medications. He also drank 10 to 12 mugs of coffee every day just to be "functional."

He described his symptoms as being sad and not laughing, having difficulty socializing, and feeling tired, exhausted, having no emotions, having no joy with his friends or girlfriend. He denied any suicidal thoughts, history of suicide attempts or hospitalization.

He said he'd never had manic or panic attack symptoms, any obsessive/compulsive behavior, any paranoia, delusions or hallucinations. He had no medical problems, and did not take any medications or over-the-counter drugs.

On a scale of 1 to 10, 10 being the best and 1 being the worst, Tom's overall functioning at work is between "7" to "8" but only a "2" at home and in social settings. His personal and sexual relationship with his girlfriend, with whom he has been living for four years, is between "1" and "2." Likewise, on the same scale, 10 having no depression and 1 being the worst, he describes himself as being "around 2."

Tom described his current stressors as his depression and financial problems. His support is limited despite being raised in this area. His strengths include having a good job and being in good health otherwise.

Based upon these findings, my diagnostic impression for Tom was Major Depressive Disorder, recurrent, Alcohol Dependence, and relationship issues.

Tom was not using any precautions in his sexual adventures. He had no prior homosexual experiences. I expressed my concerns about HIV infection. He was not as concerned. I gave him the name of an Indian physician to get a thorough physical examination, along with blood work to make sure that he does not pass on any infection to his girlfriend. Further, I also expressed concerns with his Master-Slave relationship, and urged him to seek psychotherapy. Names of male therapists were given to him. Regarding his depression, I started him on Wellbutrin and set a follow up appointment.

Tom brought to the next session a confidential note in a sealed envelop for me; it was from his Master and Tom did not know the contents. It was hand written in poor English on a white sheet of paper with lines on both sides. It stated essentially that if I wanted to have any sexual or other services performed by Tom, he would gladly do so. Further, it stated that since I was from an Eastern country, I would understand this relationship, that his sole objective was to teach Tom different types of sex so that he could get over his inhibitions.

I was shocked. I asked Tom if I could make a copy of the note and keep it in the chart. He did not agree. I gave him the note back in its envelop for his Master without any comment.

Tom denied any suicidal thoughts and said he felt no threat of harm from Master or his friends.

Even on the Wellbutrin, there was no change in his depression. I increased it gradually from 200 mg per day to 400 mg. He did not seek help for counseling. Also, he had not made an appointment to see Dr. Shah. I again urged him to use proper precautions.

We set a return appointment for two weeks later. Tom never showed up.

CHAPTER 26

High School Dropout: A Successful Banker

I not only have my secrets, I am my secrets.

And you are your secrets …

Trusting each other enough to share them with each other

Has much to do with the secret of what it is to be human.

Frederich Buechner

Audrey is a 5-foot-10, attractive blond who has the presence of a movie star. She is in her late 40s, but her looks defy her age; she appears at least 10 years younger. Her voice is soft with polite manners. She commands attention. Wherever she goes, people admire her beauty, her clothes, her near perfect makeup.

She is a successful banker.

But she has numerous secrets.

She can hide her depression very well. She's been having suicidal thoughts since she was a child, though she's never acted on them. She never shows her emotions in public; she smiles always and you cannot make out what she is thinking. She cries a lot, but only at night in her bedroom with the doors locked. Her boyfriend has no clue that she is depressed; he does not even know she's seeing a psychiatrist.

There's more. She plucks eyelashes and hair from her head and pubic area; she wears a wig to cover the bald spots.

She has genital herpes that she got from a relationship.

She is a control freak. She keeps every thing in perfect order, because she is a perfectionist.

She was sexually abused by her father from the age of 10 to 12.

Though she gives the impression that she may have gone to an Ivy League school, she's actually a high-school dropout.

She gave up a daughter for adoption when she was only 16 years old.

About 10 years ago, Audrey sought help for her depression from her primary care physician, who treated her with Prozac, Zoloft, and Wellbutrin. She took these drugs for several years but was not getting well, so she very reluctantly sought help from a psychiatrist who worked with a psychologist in the same office. The psychologist diagnosed her with Attention Deficit Disorder along with depression, and she was treated by the psychiatrist with Celexa and Adderall. These helped with depression and attention problems, but her hair-pulling became worse. She took these medications for only six months.

Audrey was referred to me by her best friend, who is my patient.

When she came to my office in November 2002, she was taking Provigil for idiopathic CNS hyper somnolence (excessive day time sleepiness), prescribed by a neurologist, and Acyclovir for herpes.

Audrey was crying a lot, feeling depressed and irritable, missing work, feeling distracted and not focused at her job, having difficulty dealing with her job and customers. She described her lifelong obsessions of keeping things in order, being in control, plucking her hair. She also had premenstrual symptoms that lasted for five to seven days each month.

She denied any history of abusing alcohol or drugs. She doesn't smoke cigarettes and drinks wine only socially. She said she didn't feel paranoid, delusional or have hallucinations.

On a scale of 1 to 10, 1 being the worst and 10 being the best, she described her overall functioning at work, home, and social settings at around 4, 1, and 3, respectively. On the same scale, 10 having no symptoms and 1 being the worst, she described her depression, ADD, and OCD symptoms to be around 3, 4 and 5.

Audrey was born into an upper middle class business family in Charleston, S.C. She had a good childhood -- except that she was physically, emotionally and sexually abused by her father for several years. She has an older brother and a younger sister. She gets along well with them. Her mother is alive; her father died at the age of 62. Her mother has a history of depression, and both parents had bad tempers.

Audrey got pregnant at 16, dropped out of high school, and gave up her daughter for adoption. She got married at the age of 17 and was married for eight years. She has a grown-up daughter who suffers from OCD. She was married for the second time at the age of 35; this relationship lasted five years. She has a 12-year-old daughter who suffers from Bipolar Disorder. She has been divorced for seven years and is in a relationship with a 52-year-old banker.

Audrey has worked in banking for over 20 years and is now a senior vice president. She took college courses on the side, along with professional enhancement courses. She is extremely competitive, and climbed the ladder of corporate banking with charm and hard work.

I diagnosed her with Major Depressive Disorder, Obsessive Compulsive Disorder, Trichotilomania (pulling of hair), and Attention Deficit Disorder.

I gave her a prescription for Wellbutrin and told her to continue taking the Provigil.

Two weeks later, Audrey was taking the Wellbutrin 100 mg twice daily, and her depression had started to improve. She was not crying as much. She had no sexual or other side effects. There was no improvement in her OCD symptoms, however. She was started on Prozac 20 mg, and her dose of Wellbutrin was increased gradually to 400 mg daily.

Meanwhile, she went to see her neurologist, who increased her Provigil to 200 mg twice daily.

With the combination of Prozac and Wellbutrin, her mood improved significantly. She was more focused in her work, less forgetful, less irritable. She was further astonished that her hair-pulling, which she has been doing since age 8, reduced drastically. She had no side effects from the medications.

In the New Year, conflicts rose from all corners. Audrey reported conflict at work with a new supervisor. Her teenage daughter had started acting out and was not doing well in school. Her daughter switched to a new child psychiatrist who changed her medications. They moved to a bigger house. These stressors caused strain in her relationship with her boyfriend.

This was all too much for this single mother. I recommended that she seek individual and family psychotherapy as soon as possible.

I increased the dose of Prozac to 40 mg along with Wellbutrin 400 mg. Since she had done so well on this combination, she started taking Provigil only as needed.

Despite the psychosocial stressors, her psychiatric symptoms stabilized, except for problems with focus and attention. Since she had side effects from Adderall, I started her on Strattera and asked her to discontinue Provigil.

With these adjustments in medications (Prozac 40 mg, Wellbutrin 400 mg, and Strattera 40 mg), and psychotherapy, Audrey's psychiatric symptoms came under control. She had no side effects. She started to do regular exercise. She had more energy to handle conflicts at work and at home.

I continue to see her once every one or two months.

CHAPTER 27

My Wife Is Cheating On Me

Anyone who has ever struggled with poverty knows
How extremely expensive it is to be poor.
James Baldwin

Brian was 47 years old when he came to see me. His primary care physician referred him. Brian complained that his wife was cheating on him. He was unemployed after losing his high-paying job as vice president of a trucking company. He is very depressed, having episodes of crying and tearfulness. He's lost weight and has no appetite. He's irritable and is fighting with his wife. He thinks his 16-month-old son Jason is not his child. He is paranoid; people are talking about him, and they don't like him.

Brian is a racquet ball champion. His wife, Margie, is a marathon runner. She travels on her own to different races in the country. She is 12 years younger than Brian. They have been married for three years.

Brian says for several years his depression has been cyclical, lasting for two to four days once a month. But since he lost his job, the depression doesn't go away. Over the past weekend Brian had severe feelings of hopelessness, helplessness and being empty, "wanting to end it all." He denied any current thoughts of suicide, plan or intent. He also denied any previous history of suicide attempt or hospitalization in a psychiatric hospital. He said he had no guns at home.

Brian used to drink two to four cocktails a day, sometimes more. But for three months, he has stopped drinking and has been going to AA meetings. He is on his fourth step of the 12-step recovery process.

Brian was first married at 23. About 10 years ago, he had extensive psychotherapy for a year, when he got divorced from his first wife, who ran away with his best friend and took his Mustang. His parents died around that same time.

He is currently on unemployment benefits. He's stressed about having lost his job and looking for another one, the conflict at home, and his depression becoming worse.

Six weeks ago, his primary care physician prescribed him Lithium Carbonate 300 mg twice daily. He doesn't want to take this medication, and was thus referred to my office.

Brian's mother used to suffer from depression. She died of cancer at the age of 59. His father was an engineer. He used to drink heavily, and there is a history of drinking in his side of the family. He died at the age of 64 of cancer. Brian's older brother is a drug addict and alcohol abuser, and he has been in and out of psychiatric hospitals. His two younger brothers drink heavily, and a younger sister suffers from depression.

Born and raised in Long Island, New York, Brian had one year of college. He describes his family as dysfunctional. His father was a pathological liar and a heavy drinker. His mother was

Catholic and went to church every Sunday. Brian is emotionally like his father. He was gifted as a trumpet player. He played in school bands, and once in Carnegie Hall. He also has a certification for piano repair. His relationship with his siblings is distant. He did not talk to his parents or family for more than 10 years. He was not invited to his sister's wedding, and at his mother's funeral, there was no chair for him.

Brian was an athlete with good looks, and he was able to "sell" things successfully, but he had difficulty sticking with the job due to his personality conflicts with coworkers or supervisors. Because of that he was usually either promoted or fired. Most of his adult life he worked in the trucking industry.

My diagnosis was Major Depressive Disorder with Psychotic features, History of Alcohol Dependence, and marital problems. I discontinued the Lithium and started him on Haloperidol 1 mg, and Prozac 20 mg per day. We discussed a "No Harm" contract, and I told him that he was to call my office or go to the hospital should his suicidal thoughts get out of control.

At the next session, Brian reported that he was not feeling as rejected or paranoid. His depression was also improving, as well as his functioning. He had no side effects from the medications. He was playing racquet ball, and had mild stiffness of his muscles. He had no interview for a job. I increased his Haloperidol to 1.5 mg, and gave him a prescription of Cogentin (benztropin) 1 mg for any side effects, as needed. A return appointment was given in three weeks.

I got a call from Margie that Brian was having violent rages. He had thrown dirty underwear at her and had grabbed her arms and face.

We do take information from family or other sources who call us. But we do not give any information about patients to others without explicit written permission. Thus, I told Margie she could ask Brian to come early or she could come with him so that we could discuss the issues and the progress. Further, I recommended marital therapy.

Privacy of medical information has become a big issue in the medical legal arena. New laws of HIPPA have been instituted, and all medical practices have to comply, otherwise they are fined heavily. Legal and regulatory professionals are salivating to make money from the so-called rich, unethical doctor's practices that are not compliant with these regulations. Doctors are under the gun to comply and hold the highest ethical standards among all professionals. Sometimes a professional life is ruined over minor infractions.

At the next session, Brian reported 95% improvement in his mood and paranoid thinking. He had stopped taking Prozac, and had no side effects of stiffness of muscles from Haloperidol. He had several interviews but did not get the job. He denied any further incident of abuse to his wife, and said his rages were also subsiding. He felt more upbeat and optimistic. A return appointment was given in six weeks.

Brian described continuous positive growth in his personal relationship with Margie and their son Jason. He was communicating better. He was not feeling paranoid or delusional. His depression and rages were gone, and there was no verbal or physical abuse. Regarding alcohol, he stated that he had no need for it. He still had no job. Due to satisfactory progress, I reduced his Haloperidol to 1 mg, and gave a return appointment in two months.

At this session, Brian was feeling depressed as his unemployment benefits were cut off and he had no job. He started looking for a clerical job at a lumber or grocery store. He also started going to AA meetings again. He was getting along well at home. He complained of having no sexual desire for a long time, and having no erection in the morning on waking up. His paranoia, delusions and rages were significantly diminished. His relationship with his son and wife were improving. I continued Haloperidol and added Wellbutrin 75 mg twice daily to see whether this improved his sex life.

Within two weeks Brian called that he was getting anxious on Wellbutrin, and wanted 10 mg of Prozac. Further, he had lost his medical insurance and was unable to come to my office.

Brian finally returned after three months. He was taking only 1 mg of Haloperidol. He had been working at $7 per hour at a grocery store. He had no problems with mood, paranoid thinking, delusions or phobias. He was maintaining his sobriety and going to AA meetings. He again complained of sexual problems. In addition to Haloperidol, I prescribed Yohimbine.

Two months later, Margie and Brian came together. Brian had gotten a job with a national trucking company. He had medical insurance, and he was happy. Margie was concerned about the fact that he was drinking one or two beers per day and said that they both had a low sex drive, despite seeing pornographic movies. Yohimbine did not help. I recommended they see a sex therapist.

At the next session in a month, Brian was not concerned about sex anymore. He was not happy with the job, as his experience was not being fully utilized, but to his surprise, he was getting along better with coworkers and not taking things personally as he used to. He was more relaxed. He started playing racquet ball again, and his wife was going to the YMCA. He had no side effects from the medications.

I continued to see Brian once every two to three months. He got a job as Director of Sales and Marketing with another trucking company with a business of over $ 20 million per year. Margie became pregnant and delivered a healthy baby boy, David, in June 1996.

Brian made an interesting observation that if he reduced the Haloperidol to 0.5 mg, he started feeling paranoid within 3 days; at 1 mg he had no paranoia; and at 1.5 mg his obsessions and phobias were reduced.

All along I offered Brian the possibility of switching Haloperidol to second generation antipsychotic medications with lesser side effects. Initially he was reluctant due to cost and a higher co-payment. Now that he had a good job and better insurance, he was switched to Risperdal.

On this medication Brian had less grogginess in the morning. He took this medication for six months, and then he wanted to go back on Haloperidol because he was having problems with gas and vomiting. I had no objection to the change. I continued to see Brian once every three months.

On Wellbutrin SR, he developed a rash and thus it was discontinued. This helped to reduce his smoking, but did not help with his sex drive. Viagra also did not help.

Brian has been happy with his job and family. He has gotten several promotions at work. This is the first time in his life that he has been stable at his job for several years. He plays golf instead of racquet ball to entertain his clients. He's still drinking two to three beers daily, and Margie is still critical of his drinking, but they get along well. They go to their childrens' games and PTA meetings at school. Brian is stable on Risperdal 2 mg, and Celexa 20 mg. I continue to follow him once every two to three months.

Brian's story, like many others, is a good example of how regulated managed care and skyrocketing malpractice insurance premiums have affected doctors. Doctors face a true dilemma when their patients lose their jobs or insurance or when they otherwise cannot pay their fees. In the past, I used to reduce or forgive charges. But with managed care, the insurance rates of doctors' fees are reduced by 30% to 40% of the customary rates. Further, insurance companies delay payments or put hurdles in the paying process. Small practices that cannot afford more staff either give up or forgive the amount, which, of course, becomes profit for the insurance company. I do not know of any other profession where accounts receivable is so difficult and cumbersome. This is exactly the reason why many doctors cannot afford to start their own practice. Thus more and more solo practices are disappearing, and the practice of medicine is becoming a corporate business.

Financially, there is no guarantee of payment for doctors' services. Nearly every other service in the world is guaranteed payments, and no one hassles with the rates. Not true for a physician. For example, attorneys can charge $200 to $800 per hour, a plumber can charge $50 to $75 per hour, and no one dare ask a question about the bills. Doctors' earnings have decreased over the past 10 years due to managed care and escalating malpractice insurance premiums. And there is no distinction between the best and the worst, or between the least and most experienced doctors, as they are paid the same. Thus, the best brains are not going into medicine. There is a national crisis.

Another alarming development related to money is the fact that the Mental Health Center Act of 1964 is being dismantled due to budget cuts at the state level. This act mandated all states to have mental health centers to provide psychiatric care to the mentally ill. These centers are being converted to financially self-supported businesses. That means that even indigent patients have to pay for the services, and these places will have to compete for business with private practices that do not get any subsidies from the local, county or state governments. As a consequence of this drastic change in the policy, many mental health professionals, such as therapists, psychologists, case workers, substance abuse counselors, marriage and family therapists -- and even psychiatrists -- are going to lose their jobs. That means more mentally ill people are going to be in jails or on the streets.

CHAPTER 28

Death Of An Addict

Every form of addiction is bad,
No matter whether the narcotic be
Alcohol or morphine or idealism.
Carl Jung

Jack was always at the top of his class. He was intelligent and fun loving, a risk taker. He helped his father in the construction material business even in high school. His father, realizing his potential, used to give him plenty of money. He was a favorite child of his mother. He used to tell her everything. His vices, even in high school, were drugs and loose women. He started abusing alcohol and marijuana at parties in high school.

Jack's 46-year-old brother, Ted, who is three years older, went to North Carolina State University and majored in business. Jack followed in his footsteps. They enjoyed doing hard drugs, such as cocaine and heroin. Their younger brother, Ben, graduated from UNC Chapel- Hill; he did not do drugs. They all joined the family business. With a boom in construction over the past 20 years in this area, they built the business from $10 million per year to $100 million per year.

Jack has been married for 15 years. He and his wife, Ann, have been having marital problems. Ann is two years younger and does not work outside the home. They have two daughters, ages, 14 and 8.

Jack was referred by a friend from college, who is also my patient, and came to see me in December 2000. Ann had decided to terminate the marriage. Jack had sought help of a private detective last year, and there was a possibility of involvement with another man. Recently, she had moved to another bedroom in the house. He wanted to know how to tell the children about their problems.

Jack was feeling very depressed, tearful, withdrawn, and anxious. He was not eating, and thus losing weight, and not thinking clearly. These symptoms had persisted for nearly two months and were getting worse. It was beginning to affect his business.

Jack's depression started in his early 20s. He has been under the care of psychiatrists since then. He has been on Elavil, Wellbutrin, Zoloft and Prozac in the past. About a week ago he started back on Prozac. He was on antidepressants about a year ago.

He denied any suicidal thoughts or attempts or history of hospitalization in a psychiatric hospital. However, he was hospitalized for a crack cocaine addiction in a drug treatment facility for 28 days in 1991. He shared a significant history of marijuana and opioids abuse, including heroin in 1995. He says he's off all illicit drugs and over-the-counter medications, but he chews 12 Nicorette 4 mg gum pieces a day, equivalent to at least two packs of cigarettes, and drinks five 12-ounce bottles of Mountain Dew containing lots of caffeine.

Jack, who's 6 feet tall, has been physically healthy except for minor hypertension, which is controlled with a medication.

There is a history of depression and alcohol abuse in both grandfathers. His sister suffers from depression.

Jack described his current stressors as the marriage problems and the fact that his father was dying of asbestosis and had to be on oxygen all the time.

I gave a diagnosis of Major Depressive Disorder, recurrent, Caffeine and Nicotine Dependence, History of Polysubstance (marijuana, cocaine, opioids) dependence, and marital conflicts. I increased his Prozac to 40 mg, and strongly recommended psychotherapy.

Two weeks later, Jack stated that he had not been feeling as dark and depressed. His wife was still sleeping in a separate bedroom. He had a good Christmas with his family and children. He said he was having difficulty accepting the separation, even though he has been involved with another woman, Paula, on the side, for at least 10 years. He complained of problems with erection. He lost another four pounds.

He came one week earlier than his scheduled appointment. He complained of being more depressed, sleeping too much, and feeling very tired. He described being torn in the marriage. He had been putting all his assets together for a separation agreement. I reduced his Prozac and started him on Wellbutrin. He was strongly advised again to see a psychotherapist as soon as possible.

Jack did well on the Wellbutrin. His usage of Nicorette gum reduced from 12 to eight per day. Likewise, his need for caffeinated drinks also started to subside. He started seeing a therapist, and also planned to go for mediation to finalize the separation agreement with his wife. His parents and brothers were aware of his problems, and they had taken over his responsibilities in the business. He had taken some Valium from his sister-in-law and said it helped with anxiety.

The separation agreement was finalized with the help of an attorney, and the children were told. They had a hard time accepting the separation. Jack moved out of the house and rented an apartment not far away. He invited his friend Paula to come and live with him. He did not tell the children about Paula.

Paula had a strong history of heavy drug abuse. She had been through many drug rehabilitation programs and community mental health centers all her adult life. She had lived with many different men who could provide shelter for her. She was also addicted to alcohol and over-the-counter pills containing caffeine and ephedrine. She had never held onto a job. She was totally dependent on Jack.

Jack had a special affinity for Paula because they'd known each other for so long. He decided to ease the pain of his separation by asking her to move in, but he was actually adding another huge responsibility that he was not ready for. She cleaned his apartment and provided him sex and drugs. He was back into opioids and cocaine.

Jack heard of a drug rehabilitation program in the Caribbean Island of St. Kitts, offered by the Healing Visions Institute for Addiction Recovery, conducted by a famous addiction pharmacologist-scientist, Deborah Mash, Ph.D., professor at the University of Miami, Fla. They are conducting trials with a plant alkaloid, Ibogaine for addiction cessation from opioids, alcohol and cocaine. This treatment is not approved by the FDA in the United States. It costs about $15,000 for a two-week program.

Jack, without my input, enrolled into this program and went off all medications for depression, as required by the protocol.

When he came back from the Caribbean by the end of July 2001, he had been off of Wellbutrin, Nicorette gum and his blood pressure medication. He was relaxed and his mood was better. He was warned that he may go into depression after three to six months. Paula was still living with him, but the separation papers were not signed. He was frustrated, but he resumed his full responsibilities at work. He wanted Viagra for his erection problems.

After two months of sobriety, he was legally separated in September. Gradually he started drinking alcohol, and becoming intoxicated over the weekends. He denied abusing cocaine or opioids.

Besides being sexually involved with Paula, he started seeing other women. His need for Viagra increased. Unfortunately, he stopped seeing the therapist.

The mixture of excessive alcohol and sex tipped his emotional equilibrium into depression within a month. I started him on Prozac, which he did not like, then went back to Wellbutrin.

Over holidays, Jack's depression took a deep dive. Paula was still living with him, and his children did not know about her, thus they could not come to visit him. He felt disgusted about Paula's drinking, addiction to caffeine and ephedrine and heavy smoking. He did not know what to do. I added Effexor to the Wellbutrin to see if his depression would ameliorate. I strongly recommended that he see the therapist as soon as possible.

Effexor did not help. It made him a zombie, so it was discontinued. Jack's depression was becoming worse. He was not sleeping and had a poor appetite. I gave him samples of Remeron and Paxil to add to the Wellbutrin dose. His frustrations with Paula were making him more depressed. Also, he got the bad news that his brother -- who had been sober for several years – had started abusing cocaine again. He remained sober despite these problems and strong temptations.

In early February 2002, Paula overdosed on numerous pills. 911 was called, and from the E.R. she was sent to the state psychiatric hospital about 80 miles away. Jack went to see her several times. I strongly advised that after her discharge from hospital, Paula should go somewhere else rather than coming back to him. He had a hard time exercising a tough love approach. He was earnestly addicted not only to drugs but to Paula as well.

Finally he started seeing the therapist who had helped him with his separation papers.

During Paula's absence, Jack started abusing heroin, and he stopped going to work.

Paula was discharged from the state hospital to her aunt's home, where she was not comfortable. So Jack brought her back to his place. She kept the apartment clean and was sober. She continued on her medications. Jack responded to the higher dose of Effexor XR 150 mg three times a day, along with 400 mg of Wellbutrin, and he stopped abusing drugs.

His father passed away in the spring, and Jack offered the eulogy at the church.

He was feeling better. He was productive at work.

Paula did well for six to eight weeks, then started abusing drugs again. Jack was stressed. She stole all his medications.

He bought a new house and did not want to tell Paula where he was moving. He changed his telephone number. This strategy worked for two months. He felt great. He was back at work full time. He started seeing other women. Except for social drinking, he denied abusing drugs. I strongly recommended that now, as he was relatively clean, he should start a new life of going to AA/NA meetings and get a sponsor. Further, I urged him to get an HIV test, along with a complete physical examination.

In September, Jack reported that Paula was coming back to his life. His mother, to whom he has been open and honest, was very disappointed. However, he made arrangements with a church-based program for rehabilitation where Paula was committed for a year. This was a good compromise. They could still see each other, but there was no physical contact, and she could not use any drugs.

Jack continued to make satisfactory progress. He had a good Christmas and New Year. He was back to work full time. His depression was under control with Wellbutrin and Effexor. He was traveling on business. He was dating other women. He denied abuse of drugs. I continued to see him once a month.

Jack's last session was in the first week of March 2003. He had no complaints. He denied abuse of alcohol, cocaine or opioids. He had been sober for three months. It was an achievement. His mood was the best. He was functioning at his job with 100% capacity. He had no side effects from medications.

Jack did not show up for his following appointment a month later. It was unusual, as he had always been compliant with his sessions. I was not concerned. Patients sometimes forget their appointments, and when they are short on medications, they call and make a new one.

By the end of April, Jack's friend, who referred him to my office over two years ago, came for his scheduled appointment. He told me that Jack had died of a blood clot in San Diego, California, two weeks earlier. I felt awfully saddened and shocked.

Drug and alcohol dependence are brain-based illnesses. It is estimated that 12 million Americans abuse alcohol and illicit drugs, costing the United States $150 billion per year in lost productivity. Besides the stigma, the addict suffers from cravings, addiction, and withdrawals, not to mention the psychosocial stress on family and society, as well as violence and homicide, and the physical ailments associated with such addictions.

Wellbutrin has been used successfully to reduce smoking. ReVia (Naltrexone) has been useful for some individuals to reduce the cravings for alcohol. Methadone is a current treatment for heroin and opiate dependence. Unfortunately, these are not cures, only substitutions for the illicit drug. In this regards, Ibogaine or its metabolite may have an application.

It is ironic that insurance companies are not approving prescriptions of Wellbutrin or nicotine patches for smoking cessation. They are willing to pay later for smoking related illnesses which cost thousands of dollars, but not for prevention of smoking. There is something wrong with our medical system that only pays for treatment, but not for prevention. Even the medical establishment at the medical schools does not have a Department of Preventive Medicine to teach medical students and residents.

It is unfortunate that drug companies are not aggressively developing anti-addiction medications. It could be that the majority of people who suffer are from the lower socioeconomic strata of the society, people who cannot afford treatment or the cost of drugs. Further, the insurance companies are not paying for the treatment of drug rehabilitation programs, and only very well-off people can afford to go to such programs.

The model of the 28-day drug rehabilitation program has been abandoned because insurance companies refuse to pay. They only pay for very short detoxification treatment, for few days in the hospital. Thereafter, an intensive outpatient program of two to four hours in the morning or in the evening three to four times per week has also not been successful. Getting these intensive outpatient programs approved from the insurance companies has been a challenge. Due to under-funding of such programs, many treatment facilities have folded in the new environment of managed care. Unfortunately, the alcohol and drug addicts have suffered the most.

CHAPTER 29

Doctor Jay's Story

Jay had a wonderful childhood. His father was a banker and his mother was a school teacher. He was a very good student and enjoyed learning new things. After high school, Jay had no problems getting into the Computer Science Program at NYU. While working as a research lab technician in the Department of Neurology and Neurosciences at Albert Einstein Medical School in New York City, he became intrigued by the complexity of the brain and the advances in research and decided to go to medical school to pursue this fascination. He scored very high on his MCAT examination and got good recommendations from the researchers in the department. Before starting medical school, he married his high school sweetheart, Ann. They had three children, and Jay became a doctor and started a private practice in North Carolina.

He had everything going for him, but before long, he would lose it all.

THE LONG JOURNEY DOWN

When Jay first came to see me, he was 46 years old. He walked with a limp, the result of a motor vehicle accident that occurred when he was 16, one that left him needing a hip replacement with constant pain. He had been under the care of a psychiatrist at the local mental health center and had been taking 20 mg each of Zyprexa and Prozac for a few months. He had gained 20 pounds, was not sleeping well and still felt depressed. He did not feel well. He had been functioning at about 60% of his capacity. He had been suffering from mood swings and going into depression – not as severe as earlier in his life, but troubling.

Jay says his mood swings started in college. For seven to 10 days at a time, he would isolate himself and work in the library or in the lab alone. He would sleep a lot and not feel that he was working to the best of his potential. He would then get spurts of energy that lasted for one to two weeks; he'd finish all his assignments and feel at his best. He didn't think there was anything wrong with him. Jay knew that his father and grandfather had suffered mood swings as well. They were successful in what they did, so his mood swings didn't bother him.

He did not use any drugs in college.

Medical school wasn't hard for Jay -- except for dealing with his mood swings. The excitement of new knowledge and the well-disciplined schedule he kept with his supportive friends kept him away from going into deep depression. He also had excellent support from his parents and his wife.

While doing a Psychiatry rotation for two months in his senior year of medical school, Jay thought that he may be Bipolar, but he dismissed it – probably because the cases he was seeing at the hospital were extreme, and he wasn't like them. As many medical students are, Jay felt immune to his own illness; after all, he knew a lot more than many people, he was functioning well and making good grades.

Jay finished his residency training in neurology from Duke University Medical Center, and did a Fellowship in Pain Management. He also spent a year at the National Institutes of Health in Bethesda to do research in neurological disorders.

When the stress at home, work and at the hospital got to him, he had become seriously depressed. His wife was unhappy in their marriage. Jay was a social drinker in college and medical school. In his early 30s, he started drinking wine at night to get better sleep. Later he began a downward spiral of drinking, suicidal thoughts, hospitalizations. Six years ago, he overdosed on over-the-counter medications in an attempt to kill himself. He was placed in a psychiatric hospital for 10 days. He was formally diagnosed with Bipolar Affective Disorder Type 2 and treated with mood stabilizers. The following year he spent three months in an alcohol and drug treatment residential facility in Virginia. In 1998, he was hospitalized at the Mental Health Center five times and spent six weeks at the State Mental Hospital in Broughton, North Carolina. That year and the following year, he was charged with driving while under the influence of drugs or alcohol and lost his driver's license -- and his medical license.

At this critical time, his wife decided to separate. She took the children with her. Jay was heartbroken. Finally they divorced when he lost his license.

Since Jay could not work as a physician, he found a job as a computer engineer. He started going to Alcoholics Anonymous meetings for professionals. He also started seeing a therapist who treated other professionals with alcohol problems. He found a nice and caring sponsor. He also formed a solid network of trusted friends who gave him rides.

With this information on hand, I agreed with his diagnosis of Bipolar Affective Disorder Type 2, along with History of Alcohol Abuse.

Almost every state in the USA has a program to help the impaired physicians, physician assistants and their families -- to rehabilitate them from alcohol or drug abuse, sexual misconduct, untreated psychiatric illness and/or personal and family stress.

The North Carolina Physicians Health Program (NCPHP) is a non-profit organization. They have a staff of psychiatrists, physicians, physician assistants, social workers and therapists who help physicians and their families by making proper referrals for treatment. They further coordinate their efforts with the North Carolina Medical Board to restore their medical licenses.

After losing his license to practice medicine, Jay was automatically enrolled into the NCPHP. Every three months he has to get a report from his psychiatrist about his progress, submit to a urine drug screen taken at random, and meet with a counselor on a regular basis. He has been very compliant.

Jay had been treated by psychiatrists with numerous medications over the years, such as Zoloft, Paxil, Remeron, Tegretol, Depakote, Lithium, Imipramine, Wellbutrin, Effexor, Buspar, Trazodone, Ambien, Risperdal, Lamactil and Navane.

He had stopped taking Zyprexa for a week before coming to see me. Since he was not sleeping well, I started him on Trazodone and gave him a prescription of Topamax to stabilize his mood, as well as to lose weight. I also gave him a prescription of Klonopin as needed for sleep.

For patients with a history of alcohol or drug abuse many psychiatrists and physicians specialized in addiction are reluctant to prescribe medications belonging to benzodiazepine family, such as Klonopin, Valium, Librium, Ativan, Xanax or Serax. They do not want to "substitute" one addictive substance for another. Certainly, benzodiazepines have an addiction potential. But when used judiciously, and under the care of a physician, they are the safest and most effective of medications for certain problems.

Jay started to sleep better on Trazodone. He was also reluctant to take any benzodiazepines, so the Klonopin was discontinued.

When the holiday season arrived, full of Christmas parties, there was a temptation for him to drink alcohol. I suggested Naltrexone or ReVia to reduce the craving for alcohol, to which Jay agreed. The holiday season in general had been bad for him; there were lots of bad memories. His mood became tearful and sad. I started him on Wellbutrin to improve his mood and to give him better mental concentration with more energy. He responded positively to this change.

His mood swings and racing thoughts came under control with Topamax, which was gradually titrated up to 200 mg. He had no side effects. He started losing the weight he had gained on Zyprexa.

In January 2002, Jay complained of feeling paranoid and of his boss not liking him, as well as believing that people were following him. It is quite possible that he had felt this way in the past and was treated with Risperdal, Navane and Zyprexa. Based on this information, I revised his diagnosis to Bipolar Affective Disorder Type 2, with minor psychotic features. I started him on Geodone, to which he responded satisfactorily at 40 mg.

I continued to see Jay once a month. He remained compliant with his medications. He also continued to see his therapist on a regular basis. He religiously went to AA meetings. I encouraged him to go to church and other non-AA group places. He was, however, limited by his driving.

His AA sponsor, who is an attorney, helped him through the process of arranging for a hearing before the Department of Motor Vehicles to regain his driver's license. He got the license in February 2002; he was happy to have the freedom to go any place on his own and as a result was able to go to more meetings and meet more people.

During retreat meetings through his church, he met a woman and they began dating. He was quite excited as he had not dated since his divorce. He started to pay more attention to his clothes and personal appearance. He joined the YMCA to do regular exercise.

After the death of his father, his mother moved to Florida. Jay was happy that his 86-year-old mother decided to come to

Charlotte and live with him. His children, who live only an hour away, were coming more frequently to visit and were spending more time with him. His ex-wife was engaged, and she exercised less control over the children. Jay was looking more optimistically toward his future.

In order for Jay to have his medical license reinstated, he was advised by NCPHP to take some refresher courses and an internship with a mentor. He found a well-established neurologist who was willing to be his mentor. He gradually transitioned to working 50% on his job and 50% doing clinical work. He finally completed his application for restoration of his medical license. He had good recommendation letters from the NCPHP, his therapist, his sponsor and me. He went through a formal meeting with the North Carolina Medical Board, and regained his medical license.

Jay has been stable since then with the help of medications and therapy. He's currently taking Wellbutrin, Geodone, Lexapro and Trazodone. He is looking forward to his new professional and personal life. I continue to see him once every month or two.

SECTION THREE :

APPENDICES

I am of the opinion that my life belongs to the whole community, and as long as I live, it is my privilege to do for it whatsoever I can. I want to be thoroughly used up when I die, for the harder I work the more I live. I rejoice in life for its own sake. Life is no brief candle to me, but a sort of splendid torch which I have got hold of, and I want to make it burn as brightly as possible before handing it on to future generations.

George Bernard Shaw

CHAPTER 30

Common Psychiatric Disorders

Adjustment Disorders is diagnosed when psychiatric symptoms are in response to an identifiable stress or stressors within 3 months of onset.

Alcohol Abuse, Alcohol Dependence, Alcohol Intoxication, and Alcohol Withdrawal are all related to alcohol use.

Alzheimer Dementia is most common among dementia. It can be accompanied by depression, delusions, or delirium.

Amphetamine Abuse, Amphetamine Dependence, Amphetamine Intoxication, and Amphetamine Withdrawal are related to amphetamine use.

Antisocial Personality Disorder is a pervasive pattern of disregard for and violation of the rights of others since age 15 years. Prior to that in childhood, this disorder is described as **Conduct Disorder.**

Anxiety Disorders: In this family of disorders are the following: Generalized Anxiety Disorder, Social Anxiety, Panic Disorder, Agoraphobia, Obsessive-Compulsive, Posttraumatic Stress, and Acute Stress.

Attention-deficit Disorder (ADD), and Attention-deficit Hyperactivity Disorder (ADHD): The major features of these disorders are problems with attention, focus, hyperactivity, and impulsivity.

Bipolar Disorders: These disorders have at least one manic episode followed by depressive episodes. There is a huge difference in the quality and frequency of these symptoms over the life time of patients ranging from mild to very severe ones. Sometimes they are accompanied by psychotic symptoms. Patients with these symptoms may need mood stabilizers, antidepressants and antipsychotic medications.

Bulimia Nervosa: In this disorder, patients have recurrent episodes of binge eating, followed by recurrent inappropriate behavior of self-induced vomiting, abuse of laxatives, diuretics, enemas or other medications; fasting; or excessive exercise to lose weight.

Cannabis-induced Disorders are its Abuse or Dependence.

Cocaine Abuse, Cocaine Dependence, Cocaine Intoxication and Cocaine Withdrawal are related to this drug.

Cyclothymic Disorder is a milder form of Bipolar Disorder.

Delirium is disturbance of consciousness (focus, concentration, attention) and cognition (memory, disorientation, and language) developed over a short period of time.

Delusional Disorder involves symptoms of being followed, poisoned, infected, loved at a distance, or deceived by spouse or lover, or having a disease.

Depressive Disorders include Major Depressive Disorder, Single Episode, or Recurrent, as well as Dysthymic Disorder. They can be accompanied by anxiety or psychotic symptoms.

Dysthymic Disorder is a minor form of depression lasting for more than 2 years.

Eating Disorders: Anorexia Nervosa and Bulimia Nervosa are major eating disorders.

Erectile Disorder, Male is inability to attain or maintain erection until completion of sexual activity.

Gambling, Pathological is an Impulse Control Disorder.

Generalized Anxiety Disorder: In this disorder, patients have excessive anxiety and worry all the time.
Hypochondriacs: Patients with this disorder have preoccupation with fears of having a serious disease.
Impulse Control Disorders: Intermittent Explosive Disorder, Kleptomania, Pyromania, Pathological Gambling and Trichotilomania are the major disorders in this category.
Insomnia is a part of Sleep Disorders.
Intermittent Explosive Disorder is defined as discrete episodes of failure to resist aggressive impulses that result in serious assault acts or destruction of property.
Kleptomania is defined as failure to resist impulses to steal objects that are not needed for personal use or for their monitory value.
Major Depressive Disorder describes constellation of symptoms, such as depressed mood, loss of pleasure, weight loss, sleep disturbance, tiredness, no energy, reduced ability to think or concentrate, and sometimes with recurrent thoughts of suicide.

Manic Episode include symptoms of elated mood, grandiose thinking, decreased need for sleep, being more talkative than usual, racing thoughts, easy distraction, and excessive buying or making foolish business decisions.
Obsessive Compulsive Disorder is composed of recurrent and persistent thoughts, impulses or images, followed by repetitive behaviors, such as hand washing, keeping things in order, checking, praying, counting or sexually acting out.
Opioids Abuse, Dependence, Intoxication, and Withdrawal are related to opioids and their derivatives.

Oppositional Defiant Disorder describes a pattern of hostile and defiant behavior in children and teenagers.

Panic Disorder is designated when a patient experiences sudden panic attacks with symptoms of heart palpitations, sweating, shortness of breath, trembling, chest discomfort, nausea or abdominal distress, fear of losing control or dying.

Psychotic Disorders: In this category we have Schizophrenia, Schizoaffective Disorder, Delusional Disorder, and Brief Psychotic Disorder.

Schizoaffective Disorder: In this disorder there are concurrent symptoms of schizophrenia along with Major Depressive Disorder or Bipolar Affective Disorder.

Schizophrenia: In this disorder the patient experiences delusions, paranoia, hallucinations, disorganization of speech, thoughts and/ or behavior. There are several subtypes of schizophrenia, such as Paranoid, Disorganized, catatonic or undifferentiated.

Sexual Disorders: In these disorders, patients may have problems with sexual desire, sexual aversion, and sexual arousal including male erectile disorder, orgasmic, premature ejaculation, sexual pain disorder and vaginismus.

Sleep Disorders: Most common sleep problems are insomnia, hypersomnia, narcolepsy, sleep apnea and nightmares.

Social Phobia or Social Anxiety Disorder: In this disorder exposure to feared social situations invariably provokes anxiety symptoms.

Trichotilomania is recurrent pulling out of one's hair resulting in noticeable hair loss.

CHAPTER 31

Personality Disorders And Personality Styles

Personality disorders are defined in DSM IV as an enduring pattern of inner experience and behavior that deviates markedly from the expectations of the individual's culture. They are pervasive and inflexible. Their onset is in adulthood and they are stable over time; they lead to distress or impairment.

There are 10 personality disorders, and they are divided among three clusters.

Cluster A consists of the eccentric disorders, such as Paranoid, Schizoid and Schizotypal Personality Disorders. They are characterized by a pervasive pattern of abnormal cognition, self expression and interpersonal relationship.

Cluster B consists of the dramatic disorders, such as Antisocial, Borderline, Histrionic and Narcissistic Personality Disorders. They are characterized by a pervasive pattern of violating social norms, impulsivity, excessive emotionality, grandiosity or acting out.

Cluster C consists of anxious disorders, such as Avoidant, Dependent and Obsessive-Compulsive Personality Disorders. They are characterized by a pervasive pattern of abnormal fears involving social relationships, separation, and need for control.

Personality disorders are coded on Axis II in order to separate them from the major mental disorders, which are coded on Axis I. A patient may have both Axis I and Axis II diagnoses. There is an overlap of symptoms between Axis I and Axis II. Once

Axis I symptoms are treated successfully, the Axis II symptoms typically start to fade. In order to treat Axis II disorders, intensive psychotherapy along with medications become very important.

It is not easy to diagnose Axis II personality disorders. Due to overlap of symptoms, a patient may have two to three personality disorders, which can become very confusing. In order to solve this problem, Oldham and Morris in their book, "New Personality Self-Portrait" (1995, Bantam Book, New York) very elegantly defined 14 personality styles – Conscientious, Self-Confident, Dramatic, Vigilant, Mercurial, Devoted, Solitary, Leisurely, Sensitive, Idiosyncratic, Adventurous, Self-Sacrificing, Aggressive and Serious. They hypothesize that we have a mixture of multiple personality styles, and according to their 107 paper pencil tests, one can plot one's personality as a self portrait that is as personal, accurate and unique as one's fingerprint. This is true. I have used this profile personally as well as on my family members and patients in psychotherapy. This book is extremely useful in helping patients understand their personalities and thus help them to solve their interpersonal problems in family and at work. I very highly recommend this book to all students of psychology and psychiatry.

Oldham and Morris further hypothesize that there is a continuum from personality style to personality disorder. An extreme in a personality style could lead to a personality disorder. For example; Conscientious style to Obsessive-Compulsive disorder, Self-Confident style to Narcissistic disorder, Dramatic style to Histrionic disorder, Vigilant style to Paranoid disorder, Mercurial style to Borderline disorder, Devoted style to Dependent disorder, Solitary style to Schizoid disorder, Leisurely style to Passive-Aggressive disorder, Sensitive style to Avoidant disorder, Idiosyncratic style to Schizotypal disorder, Adventurous style to Antisocial disorder, Self-Sacrificing style to Self-Defeating disorder, Aggressive style to Sadistic disorder and Serious style to Depressive disorder.

This scheme is very helpful for patients and therapist to work on issues as well as on their personality disorders.

CHAPTER 32

Schools Of Psychotherapies

I.Reconstructive

A. Psychoanalysis-Sigmund Freud

B. Modifications of Psychoanalysis

1.Active analytic techniques

2.Analytic Play therapy

3.Analytic psychology – Carl Jung

4.Character analysis

5.Cognitive – Jean Piaget

6.Developmental – Erik Erikson

7.Ego Psychology

8.Object Relations

9.Self Psychology – Heinz Kohut

10.Existential analysis – Ludwig Binswanger

11.Holistic analysis – Karen Horney

12.Individual psychology – Alfred Adler

13.Transactional analysis - Eric Berne

14.Washington cultural school – Harry Sullivan and Erich Fromm

15.Will therapy – Otto Rank

C. Group Approaches

1.Orthodox psychoanalytic

2.Psychodrama – J.L.Moreno

II.Reeducative and supportive, Individual and Group

III.Client centered – Carl Rogers

A.Conditioning, behavior therapy, behavior modification

1.Aversion therapy

2.Behaviorism

3.Classical conditioning - Pavlov

4. Operant conditioning - Skinner

5.Sexual counseling – Masters and Johnson

6.Systematic desensitization – Wolpe

B.Cognitive behavior therapy – Aaron Beck

C.Family therapy

D.Gestalt

E.Logo – Victor Frankle

F.Psychobiology – Adolf Meyer

G.Zen – Alan Watts

CHAPTER 33

Psychiatric Medications

ABILIFY is a trade name for Aripiprazole. It is a second generation antipsychotic medication. It is used as a mood stabilizer.

ADDERALL is a mixture of different salts of dextroamphetamine. These salts release the active drug at different rates, and thus have longer action than the parent compound. It is used for ADHD and ADD.

ADIPEX is a trade name for phenteramine. It is used as an appetite suppressant. It belongs to the family of stimulants.

ALPRAZOLAM is a generic name for Xanax. It belongs to the family of benzodiazepines. It is used for panic and anxiety disorders. It has a short half-life, and thus acts fast.

AMANTADINE is an antiviral agent that is also useful to treat side effects of antipsychotic medications.

AMBIEN is a trade name for zolpidem, which is used as a sleeping agent.

AMITRIPTYLINE is a tricyclic antidepressant. It also has sedating properties. Its trade name is Elavil.

AMPHETAMINES are stimulants used for ADD, ADHD and narcolepsy. Dextroamphetamine belongs to this family of drugs.

ANAFRANIL is trade name for clomipramine. It is used for OCD and depression.

ARIPIPRAZOLE is generic name for Abilify. It is a second generation antipsychotic medication. It is also used as a mood stabilizer.

ASCENDIN is a sedating tricyclic antidepressant.

ANTABUSE is a trade name for Disulfiram. It is used in the treatment of alcohol dependence.

ANTICONVULSANT DRUGS such as Depakote, Tegretol, Trileptal, Lamictal, Neurontin, and Topamax are used as mood stabilizers. They are also helpful in explosive disorders.

SEROTONIN REUPTAKE INHIBITORS (SRI) such as Prozac, Paxil, Zoloft, Celexa, Lexapro and Luvox are used for depression, OCD, bulimia, PMS, panic and anxiety disorders.

ARICEPT is a trade name for Donepezil. It is used to improve memory in dementia of the Alzheimer's type.

ATARAX is a trade name for hydroxyzine. It is used for treatment of anxiety.

ATIVAN is a trade name for Lorazepam. It is a benzodiazepine, and it is used for the treatment of anxiety and panic disorder.

ATOMOXETINE is a generic name for Strattera used in the treatment of ADD/ADHD.

BENADRYL is a trade name for diphenhydramine. It is used for treatment of side effects of antipsychotic medications, and as a hypnotic and anti itch medication.

BENZODIAZEPINES are a class of compounds used for treatment of anxiety, panic, seizures and muscle relaxants, as well as hypnotics. Valium, Librium, Ativan, Klonopin, Xanax, Serax, Restoril belong to this family.

BENZTROPINE is a generic name for Cogentin. This is used to treat side effects of antipsychotic medications.

BUPROPION is a generic name for Wellbutrin. It is used as an antidepressant and for smoking cessation.

BUSPAR is a trade name for buspirone. It is used to treat anxiety.

BUSPIRONE is a generic name for Buspar. It is used as an antianxiety agent.

CARBAMAZEPINE is a generic name for Tegretol. It used as antiseizure and antimanic drug.

CELEXA is a SRI antidepressant drug. Its generic name is Citalopram.

CHLORAL HYDRATE is an old hypnotic agent.

CHLORDIAZEPOXIDE is the generic name for Librium. It is a benzodiazepine.

CHLORPROMAZINE is the generic name for Thorazine. It was developed as an antianxiety drug. It was the first antipsychotic medication proven to be effective in treatment of schizophrenia.

CIALIS is a brand name for Tadalafil. It is a male erectile dysfunction drug.

CITALOPRAM is the trade name for Celexa. It is an SRI drug.

CLOMIPRAMINE is generic name for Anafranil. It is used for treatment of depression and OCD.

CLONAZEPAM is the generic name for Klonopin. It is a benzodiazepine. It is used for anxiety, panic and seizure disorders.

CLORAZEPATE is a benzodiazepine. Its trade name is Tranxene.

CLOZAPINE is the generic name for Clozaril. It is a second generation antipsychotic drug.

CLOZARIL is the trade name for Clozapine.

COGENTIN is the trade name for Benztropin. It is used to counteract the side effects of antipsychotic medications.

CYTOMEL is triiodothryonine. It is also called T3. It is used as an adjunct to antidepressant drugs.

DALMANE is a hypnotic agent belonging to the benzodiazepine family of medications.

DEPAKOTE is trade name for Valproic acid. It is used as an antiseizure medication and mood stabilizer in mania and explosive disorder.

DESIPRAMINE is an antidepressant drug related to Imipramine. It belongs to a class of Tricyclic antidepressants.

DESYREL is a trade name for Trazodone. It was developed as an antidepressant medication. It is currently used as hypnotic agent.

DEXEDRINE is a trade name for Dextroamphetamine.

DEXFENFLURAMINE is a trade name for Redux. It is used as appetite suppressant.

DEXTROAMPHETAMINE is a stimulant that is used for ADD, ADHD and narcolepsy. Mixture of several salts of this compound is contained in Adderall.

DIAZEPAM is a trade name for Valium.

DIPHENHYDRAMINE is a generic name for Benadryl.

DISULFIRAM is a generic name for Antabuse. It is used as an aversive conditioning treatment for alcohol dependence.

DIVALPROEX is the trade name for Valproic acid. It is similar to Valproate.

DONEPEZIL is generic name for Aricept. It is used for mild to moderate impairment of dementia of the Alzheimer's type.

EFFEXOR is the trade name for Venlafaxine. It is used as an antidepressant and antianxiety drug.

ELAVIL is trade name for tricyclic antidepressant Amitriptyline.

ELDEPRYL is trade name for monoamine oxidase inhibitor Selegiline.

ESKALITH and Lithonate are the trade names for lithium salts. They are used as mood stabilizers.

EXELON is trade name for Rivastigmine. It is used for treatment of mild to moderate cognitive impairment in dementia.

FLUOXETINE is generic name for Prozac. It is an SRI drug.

FLUPHENAZINE is generic name of Prolixin. It is an antipsychotic agent.

FLURAZEPAM is generic name for Dalmane. It is used as hypnotic agent.

FLUVOXAMINE is generic name for Luvox.

GABAPENTIN is generic name for Neurontin.

GEODONE is trade name for Ziprasidone. It is a second generation antipsychotic medication. It is also used as a mood stabilizer.

HALCION is a hypnotic agent. It belongs to the benzodiazepine family of medications.

HALDOL is trade name of haloperidol.

HALOPERIDOL is generic name for Haldol. It is an antipsychotic agent.

HYDROXYZINE is generic name for Atarax and Vistaril. It is an anti-anxiety agent.

IMIPRAMINE is a Tricyclic antidepressant.

KLONOPIN is a trade name for Clonazepam. It is a long acting benzodiazepine.

LAMICTAL is trade name for Lamotrigine. It is an antiseizure drug. It is also used as a mood stabilizer.

LAMOTRIGINE is generic name for Lamictal.

LEVOTHYROXINE is generic name for synthroid.

LEXAPRO is related to SRI Celexa.

LIBRIUM is trade name Chlordiazepoxide.

LITHIUM carbonate is used as an antimanic drug.

LITHOBID is trade name for lithium.

LORAZEPAM is generic name for Ativan.

LUVOX is a trade name for Fluoxamine. It is an SRI drug.

MELLARIL is an antipsychotic medication. Its generic name is Thioridazine.

MERIDIA is a trade name for Sibutramine. It is used for weight loss.

METHADONE is used to treat opioids addiction, and chronic pain.

METHAMPHETAMINE is a generic name for Desoxyn. It is used as an appetite suppressant.

MITRAZAPINE is a generic name for Remeron.

MOBAN is a trade name for Molindone. It is an antipsychotic medication.

MODAFINIL is generic name for Provigil. It is used to treat narcolepsy and ADD/ADHD.

MOLINDONE is generic name for Mobane.

MONOAMINE OXIDASE INHIBITORS (MAO) are a class of antidepressant medications. They are not used as much in the practice of psychiatry.

NALTREXONE is generic name for ReVia. It is used to reduce the craving for alcohol.

NARDIL is a MAO inhibitor.

NAVANE is trade name for Thiothixene. It is an antipsychotic medication.

NEFAZODONE is trade name for Serzone. It is an antidepressant medication.

NEURONTIN is trade name for Gabapentin. It is an anti seizure medication.

NORPRAMIN is trade name for Desipramine. It is a Tricyclic antidepressant.

NORTRIPTYLINE is a generic name for Pamelor. It is a Tricyclic antidepressant.

OLANZAPINE is generic name for second generation antipsychotic medication Zyprexa. It is also used as a mood stabilizer in mania.

ORAP is trade name for antipsychotic medication Pimozide.

OXAZEPAM is generic name for benzodiazepine Serax.

PAMELOR is trade name for Tricyclic antidepressant Nortriptyline.

PARNATE is a MAO inhibitor.

PAROXETINE is generic name for SRI Paxil.

PAXIL is trade name for SRI Paroxetine.

PEMOLINE is generic name for Cylert used for ADD/ADHD.

PERPHENAZINE is a generic name for Trilafon. It is an antipsychotic medication.

PHENELZINE is a MAO inhibitor.

PHENOTHIAZINE is a class of antipsychotic medications.

PHENTERAMINE is an appetite suppressant. It is generic name for Ionamin, Fastin or Adipex.

PIMOZIDE is generic name for antipsychotic medication Orap.

PROLIXIN is a trade name for antipsychotic Fluphenazine.

PROMETHAZINE is generic name for Phenergan. It is used as an anti-emetic agent.

PROPRANOLOL is a beta blocker drug used in psychiatry as an anti-anxiety agent.

PROSOM is trade name for Estazolam. It is a sedative.

PROVIGIL is trade name for Modafinil. It is used for ADD/ADHD, and narcolepsy.

PROZAC is trade name for Fluoxetine. It is an SRI drug.

QUETIAPINE is generic name for Seroquel. It is a second generation antipsychotic medication. It is also used as a mood stabilizer.

REMERON is trade name for Mitrazepine. It is an antidepressant drug.

REMINYL is trade name for Galantamine. It is used in dementia of Alzheimer.

RESTORIL is trade name for Temazepam. It is used as hypnotic drug.

REVIA is trade name for Naltrexone. It is used to reduce the craving for alcohol.

RISPERDAL is trade name for Risperidone. It is a second generation antipsychotic drug. It is also used as a mood stabilizer.

RISPERIDONE is generic name for Risperdal. It is a second generation antipsychotic medication. It is also used as a mood stabilizer.

RITALIN is trade name for Methylphenidate. It is used for ADD/ ADHD.

SEROTONIN REUPTAKE INHIBITORS (SRI) are important class of medications. Prozac, Paxil, Zoloft, Celexa, Luvox, and Lexapro belong to this class of drugs.

SERAFEM is another trade name for Prozac. Its generic name is Fluoxetine.

SERENTIL is a trade name for Mesoridazine. It is an antipsychotic medication.

SEROQUEL is trade name for Quetiapine. It is a second generation antipsychotic medication. It is also used as a mood stabilizer.

SERTRALINE is generic name for Zoloft. It is an SRI medication.

SERZONE is trade name for Nefazodone. It is an antidepressant drug.

SILDENAFIL is generic name for Viagra.

SINEQUAN is trade name for Doxepin. It is a Tricyclic antidepressant.

SONATA is a trade name for Zaleplon. It is a hypnotic agent.

STELAZINE is trade name for Trifluoperazine. It is an antipsychotic medication.

STRATTERA is trade name for ADD/ADHD medication Atomoxetine.

SYNTHROID is thyroid medication.

TEGRETOL is a trade name for Carbamazepine. It is an anti-seizure medication.

TEMAZEPAM is a generic name for Restoril. It is a hypnotic agent.

THIORIDAZINE is generic name for Mellaril. It is an antipsychotic agent.

THIOTHIXINE is generic name for Navane. It is an antipsychotic medication.

THORAZINE is a trade name for Chlorpromazine. It is an antipsychotic medication.

TOFRANIL is trade name for Imipramine. It is a Tricyclic antidepressant.

TOPAMAX is a trade name for Topiramate. It is an anti-seizure medication.

TOPIRAMATE is a generic name for Topamax.

TRANXENE is a trade name for Clorazepate. It is a benzodiazepine drug.

TRANYLCYPROMINE is a generic name for Parnate. It is a MAO inhibitor.

TRAZODONE is a generic name for Desyrel. It is a hypnotic agent.

TRIAZOLAM is a generic name for Halcion. It is a hypnotic agent.

TRIFLUPERAZINE is a generic name for Stelazine.

TRILAFON is a trade name for Perphenazine.

VALIUM is a trade name for Diazepam. It belongs to the benzodiazepine family of medications.

VALPROATE is a generic name for Depakote.

VENLAFAXINE is generic name for Effexor. It is an antidepressant medication.

VIAGRA is trade name for Sildenafil. It is used for erectile dysfunction in males.

VISTARIL is a trade name for Hydroxyzine.

WELLBUTRIN is trade name for Bupropion. It is an antidepressant medication.

XANAX is a trade name for Alprazolam. It belongs to the benzodiazepine family of medications.

YOCON is trade name for Yohimbine. It is used for male sexual dysfunction.

YOHIMBINE is generic name for Yocon.

ZALEPLON is a generic name for Sonata. It is a hypnotic agent.

ZIPRASIDONE is a generic name for Geodone. It is a second generation antipsychotic medication. It is also used as a mood stabilizer.

ZOLOFT is trade name for Sertraline. It is an SRI antidepressant.

ZOLPIDEM is generic name for Ambien. It is a hypnotic agent.

ZYBAN is another trade name for Wellbutrin. Its generic name is Bupropion.

ZYPREXA is trade name for Olanzapine. It is a second generation antipsychotic medication. It is also used as a mood stabilizer.

CHAPTER 34

Brand And Generic Drugs, And Their Manufacturers

Brand Name	Generic Name	Drug Company
Abilify	Aripiprazole	Bristol-Myers Squibb/Otsuka
Adderall	Dextroamphetamine	Shire
Adipex	Phenteramine	Gate
Ambien	Zolpidem	Sanofi-synthelabo
Anafranil	Clomipramine	Mallinckrodt
Antabuse	Disulfiram	Wyeth-Ayerst
Ascendin	Tricyclic antidepressant	Lederle
Aricept	Donepezil	Pfizer
Atarax	Hydroxyzine	Roerig
Ativan	Lorazepam	Wyeth-Ayerst
Benadryl	Diphenhyramine	
Buspar	Buspirone	Bristol-Myers Squibb
Celexa	Citalopram	Forest Pharmaceuticals
Cialis	Tadalafil	Lilly
Clozaril	Clozapine	Novartis
Concerta	Methylphenidate	Alza/ McNeil
Dalmane	Flurazepam	Roche
Depakote	Valproic acid	Abbott

Brand Name	Generic Name	Drug Company
Desoxyn	Methamphetamine	Ovation Pharmaceuticals
Desyrel	Trazodone	Apothecon
Effexor	Venlafaxine	Wyeth-Ayerst
Elavil	Amitryptyline	
Eldepryl	Selegiline	Sommerset
Eskalith	Lithium carbonate	SmithKline
Exelon	Rivastigmine	Novartis
Focalin	Rexmethylphenidate	
Geodone	Ziprasidone	Pfizer
Halcion	Triazolam	Upjohn
Haldol	Haloperidol	McNeil
Klonopin	Clonazepam	Roche
Klonopin Wafers	Clonazepam	Rochc/Solvay
Lamictal	Lamotrigine	GlaxoSmithKline
Levitra	Vardenafil	GlaxoSmithKline/ Bayer
Lexapro	Escitalopram	Forest Pharmaceuticals
Librium	Chlordiazepam	Roche
Lithobid	Lithium carbonate	Solvay
Loxitane	Loxepine	Lederle
Luvox	Fluoxamine	Solvay
Mellaril	Thioridazine	Sandoz
Meredia	Sibutramine	Abbott
Metadate	Methylphenidate	Celltech
Methylin	Methylphenidate	Mallinckrodt
Mobane	Molindone	Du Pont
Nardil	Phenelzine	Park Davis

Brand Name	Generic Name	Drug Company
Navane	Thiothixene	Roerig
Neurontin	Gabapentin	Pfizer
Norpramin	Desipramine	Marion
Orap	Pimozide	Gate
Pamelor	Nortriptyline	Sandoz
Parnate	Tranylcypromine	SmithKline
Paxil	Paroxetine	GlaxoSmithKline
Prolixin	Fluphenazine	Apothecon
Prosom	Estazolam	Abbott
Provigil	Modafinil	Cephalon
Prozac	Fluoxetine	Lilly
Remeron	Mitrazepine	Organon
Reminyl	Galantamine	Janssen
Restoril	Temazepam	Sandoz
ReVia	Naltrexone	DuPont
Risperdal	Risperidone	Janssen
Ritalin	Methylphenidate	Novartis
Serafem	Fluoxetine	Lilly
Serentil	Mesoridazine	Boehringer
Serax	Oxazepam	Wyeth-Ayerst
Seroquel	Quetiapine	AstraZeneca
Serzone	Nefazodone	Bristol- Myers Squibb
Sinequan	Doxepin	Roerig
Sonata	Zaleplon	Wyeth-Ayerst
Stelazine	Trifluperazine	SmithKline
Strattera	Atomoxetinc	Lilly
Surmontil	Trimipramine	Odyssey Pharmaceuticals

Brand Name	Generic Name	Drug Company
Symbayx	Prozac and Zyprexa	Lilly
Tegretol	Carbamazepine	Novartis
Thorazine	Chlorpromazine	SmithKline
Tofranil	Imipramine	Novartis
Topamax	Topiramate	Ortho-McNeil
Tranxene	Clorazepate	Abbott
Tranxene-SD	Clorazepate	Ovation Pharmaceuticals
Triavil	Elavil and Perphenazine	Merck
Trilafon	Perphenazine	Schering
Trileptal	Oxcarbazepine	Novartis
Valium	Diazepam	Roche
Viagra	Sildenafil	Pfizer
Vistaril	Hydroxyzine	Pfizer
Vivactil	Protriptyline	Odyssey Pharmaceuticals
Wellbutrin	Bupropion	Glaxo SmithKline
Xanax	Alprazolam	Upjohn
Xanax XR	Alprazolam	Pfizer
Yocon	Yohimbine	Palisades
Zoloft	Sertraline	Pfizer
Zyban	Bupropion	Glaxo SmithKline
Zyprexa	Olanzapine	Lilly

CHAPTER 35

Private Practice Of Psychiatry

I finished my final year of residency training in psychiatry from University of North Carolina at Chapel Hill at the ripe age of 54 in 1991. I was about to start my second life as a psychiatrist.

In my first professional life, after finishing my Ph.D. in 1964, until 1984 when I went back to medical school, I was a professor, a researcher and a scientist. I had worked as a lab researcher in different fields, such as metal-ion catalysis, purification of enzymes, and elucidating their mechanisms of action, development of anti-cancer drugs, and clinical and biochemical pharmacology of anti-cancer drugs. I was familiar with the academic life of publishing scientific papers, presenting results in meetings and writing grants, as well as the politics of academia.

Through my training in behavioral sciences and psychiatry, I had come to the conclusion that it would be very hard for me to work in an organized corporate setting of academia or mental health centers. I had to be on my own in private practice. Further, my children were going to private colleges, and I needed money to support them. Thus, I started collecting all the necessary material to be ready for private practice should and when this opportunity arose.

In the academic training there are no courses for starting private practice. Either you join an existing group of private practice, or work in a corporate setting. These were the only options.

The existing group practices at that time in Charlotte were very reluctant to have me because of my different background, age, life experience, or just my personality. Therefore, I had to work out something different.

At the periphery of South Charlotte, there was a 70 bed psychiatric hospital, CPC Cedar Spring where established psychiatrists did not want to go because of distance, prestige or convenience. The administrator and the medical director offered me an opportunity to start my private practice with them. With the help of a friend who is a graphic artist, I prepared a brochure, business card and all the necessary stationary. My girlfriend, Dolores, came all the way from Texas, and with her help we bought all the furniture and decorated the office with Indian paintings. She learned the business and became office manager. We started the practice by the end of July 1991.

The hospital was referring a good number of patients, and within three to four months I became very busy.

Within a couple of years the managed care companies descended on the city, and the business part of the practice became more complicated. There were pre-approval requirements for admission to the hospital as well as to the office visit. Due to differences in insurance policies within the same company, both inpatient and outpatient benefits had to be obtained, along with the co-pays. The usual and customary fees were slashed by 40 to 50%. For hospitalized patients there were daily reviews by an MD of the insurance company with the Attending physicians. Many admissions were denied, and the hospitals and doctors were not paid for the services. Even for office visits, if there were no pre-approvals, doctors were not paid. All denied claims were direct profits for the insurance companies. Rules of medical necessity were made by the insurance companies, and not by the treating physician, although all risks of treatment were the responsibility of the clinicians. Further, only 3 to 4 outpatient visits were given for one year by some insurance companies, and in order to get more visits, an MD had to fill up a 5 to 10 page long computerized treatment plan to get additional visits; otherwise the doctors were not paid. Further restrictions were placed on how long a psychiatrist can see a patient. Generally a 15 minutes follow up visit was allowed, after the first session of 45 to 50 minutes.

With these new rules, one had only two choices: to comply with the rules, or not accept insurance business, and run the practice only on fee for service. In the first case there is an increased overhead due to the cost of running the business, but one is certainly busy. Whereas in the second case, one has to be famous or very bright to attract only self paying patients. In my experience of being in business for over 13 years, I have had no more than 15% of my patients who are self pay, the rest of them want to use their insurance for the services.

There used to be 5 psychiatric hospitals in this area until 1999. Now there are only two, one being a large community mental health center with over 30 psychiatrists. There used to be 3 large private group practices, now there is only one. Over the past 10 years, among the psychiatrists in private practice, 3 retired, 3 passed away, one committed suicide, and 16 left this area. Of these 23, only 6 new psychiatrists have come to this area. The oldest group practice in business for over 40 years with 10 psychiatrists and numerous therapists had to close. With these changes I stopped seeing patients in the hospital in 1999, and reduced my stress level by 30%. Thanks to free market competition and onslaught of managed care! Are patients and doctors happy with this system? I am not sure.

There are over 40 million uninsured Americans, and at least 10 to 20 million underinsured. Every one is afraid of losing their medical insurance. Every year the cost of medical care is going up by 12 to 14%. Thus the co-payments for visits and medications have gone up as well. The reimbursements for doctors have not kept pace with inflation, and the cost of conducting business has gone up. Something is wrong with our system of health care, despite the fact that the productivity of the American workers has increased due to proper management of mental health problems, such as depression, anxiety, bipolar, ADD, substance abuse or personal and family issues.

In the present climate, at least in this city, it is very difficult to start one's own practice due to prohibitive initial costs. One has to pay rent, furnish, buy computers and other office equipments, hire a secretary, and possibly another person to do billing, collect money, make deposits, keep accounts, pay taxes and comply with pay roll requirements, answer phone calls from patients, pharmacies, insurance companies, disability companies, lawyers, parents, spouses, emergency rooms, therapists, and be on call for 24 hours. Further, one has to be on different insurance panels to accept their patients. This is a lengthy process which may take 4 to 6 months.

The overhead costs of running a psychiatric office at maximum capacity is around 40 to 50% provided one has a stable staff with a smart office manager. I have been very fortunate to have my wife Dolores run the office. Without her help, I am not sure whether I would have survived on my own.

Based upon these observations, it seems that solo practitioners are losing grounds, and within 10 to 15 years they would disappear. Consequently there will only be large practices controlled by corporations. In this process patients are going to be the losers as the quality of doctor-patient relationship is going to erode further.

The central question is how many patients one needs to saturate a psychiatric practice. If one works 8 hours a day, and sees patient in session for 45 minutes, once a week, then the practice is saturated with 40 patients. And if one performs psychoanalysis two times per week per patient, then the practice is saturated with only 20 patients. By doing just medication check-up with supportive psychotherapy for 15 minutes with each patient, and seeing about 20 patients a day, once weekly, the practice is saturated with 100 patients. At this rate, if one sees patients once in 2 weeks, one month or two months, then the practice is saturated with a load of 200, 400 or 800 patients, respectively. And if one sees 25 patients a day, then the number of patients to saturate a practice is increased proportionately.

Of course, there are other models. Some psychiatrists see patients only for less than 10 minutes, and they have a nurse who helps the clinician to collect data, and write prescriptions. Some psychiatrists at mental health centers or even in private practice have a nurse practitioner follow patients and see them once in 4 to 6 months. Obviously there are different models of practice of psychiatry, and people are looking into cost cutting measures.

In my experience at least one third of patients drop out from the practice every year due to multiple reasons of moving, change in insurance or doctors, or just losing jobs or insurance benefits. Therefore, every psychiatrist like any other doctor needs new infusion of patients to keep the practice running.

Despite all these complications, I often ask myself a question; why I am still in business? I absolutely enjoy what I do. My happiness and satisfaction lie in the challenge to diagnose patients correctly, and target the right molecules to get them free of symptoms so that they can start functioning better. Further, I am interested in what my patients do, what their family histories are and what is their present family constellations. I want them to get out of chaos and live in harmony and peace with themselves and their environment.

I hope you have enjoyed reading these stories, and have developed a better understanding of the challenges and achievements of behavioral sciences and psychiatry.

About The Authors

V. Sagar Sethi, M.D., Ph.D. has been in the private practice of psychiatry since 1991 in Charlotte, N.C. He has a multicultural background. He was born in the state of Punjab, India. He completed his Bachelor's and Master's degree in Pharmacy as First Class First from Banaras Hindu University, Varanasi, India. He graduated with a Ph.D., Magna cum laude, from the Ludwig Maximillian University, Munich, Germany. He was a biomedical scientist at the Max-Planck Institute of Biochemistry, Munich, and at the National Institutes of Health, Bethesda, Maryland. He was a Research Associate Professor of Medicine from 1977 to 1984 at the Bowman Gray School of Medicine of Wake Forest University, Winston-Salem, N.C. He has published over 80 scientific papers in the field of biochemistry, molecular biology, pharmacology and anti-cancer drugs.

After completing medical school in Mexico, Dr. Sethi did his internship and Residency in psychiatry at the Creighton University Medical Center, and at the University of Nebraska Medical Center, Omaha, Nebraska. His final year of training in psychiatry was completed at the University of North Carolina at Chapel Hill, N.C.

Dr. Sethi is a member of several professional medical societies. He was Associate Medical Director and Chief of Staff of psychiatric hospitals.

Dr. Sethi is a United States citizen, and he has lived in the USA for over 30 years. He has traveled extensively. In addition to several other languages, he speaks German fluently.

George W. Jacobs is a writer, professor, administrator, community activist, and an ordained minister. Currently he is the Director and co-founder of the Davidson Clergy Center, Davidson, North Carolina.

Advance Praise

"Solving Psychiatric Puzzles" by V. Sagar Sethi, M.D., Ph.D., is a delightful read. The stories are fascinating and give a glimpse into the development of psychological problems as a life story. The stories themselves provide an insight into the complex nature and evolution of psychopathology. Dr. Sethi's approach to these patients and their stories, also illustrate the process by which psychiatrists can help patients.

In summary, this is a worthwhile read for patients, families, medical students, psychologists, psychiatry residents, MD's and practitioners in this field. I think the book is of great value in pointing out the need to understand the story behind the symptoms that individuals come to physicians with.

Rama Ranga Krishnan, M.D.
Professor and Chair of Psychiatry
Duke University Medical Center
Durham, North Carolina

"Solving Psychiatric Puzzles" by Dr. Sethi is a unique book: broad in scope, yet in many ways very focused and personal.

The author draws on his own background and individual experiences in explaining the art and science of psychiatry. The patients' stories offer insights into the complexities of human behavior, and provide a very rich sampling of the world of clinical psychiatry. I can't recall ever seeing a book which applied this approach to the challenge of opening the field of psychiatry to the general public.

Robert N. Golden, M.D.
Professor and Chair of Psychiatry
Vice Dean
University of North Carolina at Chapel Hill
Chapel Hill, North Carolina

"As a retired parish minister and part-time chaplain in a mental health hospital, I enthusiastically recommend 'Solving Psychiatric Puzzles' by Dr. Sethi. He has lifted the veil from the mystery of psychiatry, and given a human face to those involved with mental illness. This book fills a void that has existed too long for both professionals and the rest of us who want to help ourselves and others live a healthy and fulfilled life."

Rev. Sidney L. Freeman, Ph.D.
Unitarian Universalist Church of Charlotte
Charlotte, North Carolina

"Solving Psychiatric Puzzles", by V. Sagar Sethi, M.D., Ph.D., is a magical book. After starting with his own personal story, Dr. Sethi takes us by his side, into the private worlds of people who were, also, his patients. We are privileged to be invited into these homes, to learn of their families, histories, sufferings, and successes. These are real people, who were dealt genetic hands that put their brains at risk, instead of their hearts or lungs or other body parts. What is remarkable, in the face of great hardship, is each individual's strength, resilience, and recovery. This is, as Dr. Sethi tells us, a book of hope and healing, a book of enlightenment, a book of amazing stories indeed.

John M. Oldham, M.D.
Professor and Chairman
Department of Psychiatry
Medical University of South Carolina
Charleston, South Carolina

"Solving Psychiatric Puzzles" by V. Sagar Sethi, M.D., Ph.D., is a one-of-a-kind book that seeks to uncover the mystery of psychiatric disorders and their treatments in a very readable fashion. Written by a well-published scientist who has been in psychiatric practice for a number of years, it provides complex information in a surprisingly personal, humanistic manner. Mental illnesses are puzzles and enigmas for most people outside the field. This book helps others understand what a person suffering from a psychiatric disease goes through. While the individual stories are deeply touching, the author succeeds in offering a clear message of hope. I would strongly recommend this outstanding book to people suffering from a mental illness, their caregivers, as well as care providers (physicians, psychologists, social workers) and students.

Dilip V. Jeste, M.D.
Chair in Aging
Director, Institute for Research on Aging
Professor of Psychiatry & Neurosciences
VA San Diego Healthcare System
University of California, San Diego

Printed in the United States
22157LVS00002B/288